Jaypee Gold Standard Mini Atlas Series®

FORENSIC MEDICINE

Jaypee Gold Standard Mini Atlas Series®

FORENSIC MEDICINE

Ashesh Gunwantrao Wankhede MD
Associate Professor
Forensic Medicine and Toxicology
Indira Gandhi Govt. Medical College
Nagpur (Maharashtra)
India

JAYPEE BROTHERS MEDICAL PUBLISHERS
The Health Sciences Publisher
New Delhi | London

Jaypee Brothers Medical Publishers (P) Ltd

Headquarters
EMCA House, 23/23-B Ansari Road,
Daryaganj New Delhi 110 002, India
Landline: +91-11-23272143,
+91-11-23272703+91-11-23282021,
+91-11-23245672
e-mail: jaypee@jaypeebrothers.com

Corporate Office
4838/24, Ansari Road,
Daryaganj New Delhi 110 002, India
Phone: +91-11-43574357
Fax: +91-11-43574314
e-mail: jaypee@jaypeebrothers.com

Overseas Office
JP Medical Ltd.
83, Victoria Street, London
SW1H 0HW (UK)
Phone: +44-20 3170 8910
e-mail: info@jpmedpub.com

EU GPSR Authorised Representative
Logos Europe, 9 rue Nicolas Poussin
17000, La Rochelle, France
Phone: +33 (0) 6 67 93 73 78
e-mail: contact@logoseurope.eu

Website: www.jaypeebrothers.com
Website: www.jaypeedigital.com

Inquiries for bulk sales may be solicited at: jaypee@jaypeebrothers.com

Jaypee Gold Standard Mini Atlas Series ® Forensic Medicine

First Edition: 2008
Reprint: **2026**
ISBN: 978-81-8448-208-9
Printed in India

I dedicate my work
to my mother
Lata
and father
Gunwantrao.
Without the great encouragement,
sacrifices and assistance of my wife
Prerana and children Öshën and Tejas this
work could not have been completed

Preface

I have a strong belief that respect is the first sign of love and justice is the greatest expression of love. I also believe that doctors are the greatest lovers in the universe as they accept their patients as they are without asking for any change in their beliefs, habits; without any discrepancies in age, sex, race, caste, color and, socioeconomic status.

I began my career in medicine about twenty years back in the atmosphere where the autopsies were conducted by mortuary attendants and doctors used to finish it by just inspecting within ten minutes; teachers in forensic medicine never bothered to teach or create interest in their subject and every student used to read book of forensic medicine ten days before examination. Then I joined forensic medicine for my postgraduate studies facing little opposition from family and friends. There I worked under a man with great philosophy and tremendous knowledge, my teacher Dr AC Mohanty, the man who made me realize the importance of my subject and respect the biological variations without any rigidity of thought. It started by conducting dissection myself; examining victims referred to our department, doing histopathology myself, consulting specialist from medical faculties and forensic science, taking their assistance and discussing the cases for hours. I know there are many like me who are in need of knowledge but may not be given proper assistance. This book is a small step towards all of them.

Being a doctor and a worker in forensic medicine I take opportunity to express my love towards humanity by assisting law for justice. There are many medical practitioners, lawyers, judges, students of medical science and forensic for whom, I think this book may be helpful.

Ashesh Gunwantrao Wankhede

Messase

Philosophy

One's ideas must be as broad as Nature if they are to interpret Nature.

Puerile as such an exercise may seem, it sharpens the faculties of observation, and teaches one where to look and what to look for.

—Sherlock Holmes

In: A Study in Scarlet by Sir Arthur Conan Doyle

Acknowledgements

I am thankful to my respected teacher Dr AC Mohanty, Professor and Head, Forensic Medicine, Terana Medical College, Nerul, Navi Mumbai, for allowing me to photograph diatoms from his collection. I sincerely appreciate his constant encouragement and invaluable. suggestions.

For editing the manuscript of this book, I am thankful to Dr Shabnam Sharan, Dr Samuel Khairkar and Dr Vaibhav Lende; without their assistance, this work could not have been accomplished.

I am indebted to my friend Dr Dinesh R Sariya, Pathologist, Western Memorial Regional Hospital, Corner Brook, Newfoundland A2H2L3, Canada for his expertise in explaining and criticizing morbid pathology and histology.

I am gratefully thankful to Dr Vinod A Agrawal, Professor and Head, Forensic Medicine, Smt KN Medical College, Narhe (Ambegaon), Pune for encouragement and being always ready for extending assistance whenever required.

I am deeply concerned with the philosophy of my friend Dr Kailash U Zine, Associate Professor, Forensic

Medicine, Govt. Medical College, Aurangabad, and thankful to his contribution of photographs on gagging and erosions caused by marking nut.

Dr Sanjay Deoba Wathore, Chief Medical Officer, Mumbai Central Prison, Arthur Road Jail, Mumbai, is the only person from India who has conducted study on the blast injury. I am very much impressed by his generous attitude towards forensic medicine and thankful for contributing photographs on bomb blast injury.

I am respectfully thankful to Dr VL Deshpande, Dr LK Bade, Dr AP Dongre, Dr HT Katade, Dr AN Keoliya, Dr SD Nanandkar, Dr CR Dode, Dr PG Dixit, Dr Ghangle, Dr HV Godbole for their blessings and constant encouragement.

I am very grateful to autopsy attendants Late Bihari uncle, Late Ramesh Khote, Shri Hari Baghel, Shri Hiralal Chindale, Shri Kiran Manpia, Shri Ramesh Dharod, Shri Bhanu Meshram, Shri Umate and Shri Gurudayal for assistance in morbid forensic medicine and for teaching me the humanitarian aspects of autopsies.

I am thankful to laboratory staff Shri Pramod Mandekar, Shri Sudesh Rathod, Shri Sunil Malke, Shri Bhaisare, Shri Vijay Indurkar and Shri Dilip Dhoke for always being available for laboratory work.

I am indebted to my undergraduate students and their parents who made me feel that I am a good teacher.

Contents

Part I: Morbid Forensic Medicine

Part II: Clinical Forensic Medicine

Part I
Morbid Forensic Medicine

1 Introduction to Morbid Forensic Medicine

Forensic medicine is a branch of medical science (other branches, e.g. anatomy, physiology, biochemistry, pathology, medicine, pediatrics, surgery, etc.) which deals with application of medical knowledge to assist law for the administration of justice. So it's all about justice 'the greatest expression of love and humanity'. When we stand as a witness before the honorable judge we proceed with oath "I swear by the almighty God, that in this evidence I shall tell the truth, the whole truth and nothing but the truth". We can understand from the oath itself that this is all about truth and not merely about the findings which we have recorded while practicing medicine. Truth is something which is beyond our findings. It may be an opinion which is drawn from the findings based on our knowledge and experience. Hence to assist law for administration of justice we must have tools of knowledge and experience.

MORBID FORENSIC MEDICINE

This branch of forensic medicine deals with dead bodies, human remains and autopsies. It is advisable to every medical student to participate or assist the residents or teachers of forensic medicine in autopsies in their undergraduate teaching program and internship. It is not just to learn forensic medicine but to learn about the human body. The body for autopsy is absolutely different from what we might have dissected in anatomy. It is not fixed by any chemical; it is exactly like a live body, but without life. It is essential to know how the heart feels in our hand; how an atherosclerotic plaque feels; how the crepitus of lung feels; how the firmness of a liver or spleen and softness of the brain feels; how the sections of a injured brain look, whether they are similar to the CT scan of head of the same person in life, etc.

This branch basically deals with application of medical knowledge to infer cause, mode, manner and mechanism of death. It also deals with matters related with identity and time since death. These are the matters in which law agencies, investigating agencies, statisticians for research, judiciary, and agencies for compensation have keen interest. Hence meticulous recording of the findings and their interpretation are demanded. This is also helpful to the medical practitioner in the witness box for answering both the counsels and remaining a man of science.

The second important part of this branch is preservation of samples for the required investigations, e.g. chemical analysis, toxicological analysis, biological study, biochemical analysis, histological study, ballistic study, entomological study, botanical study, etc.

The medical practitioner who is conducting autopsy must not only be concerned with the dead body but he must give thought to the mourners. In a country like India where people of different religions, castes and tribes live, the medical practitioner is supposed to give thought to their belief and practices of last rituals. The unnecessary delay in autopsy must be avoided and mourners must be relieved as early as possible.

2 Identification

Identification of the deceased is the sole responsibility of the investigating agency. However on receipt of the dead body and requisite papers from investigating agency, identity of every dead body must be verified by the autopsy conducting medical practitioner before beginning the autopsy. It has many advantages, like, it confirms that the autopsy of the body being conducted is the same as the one mentioned in the papers. It also gives us a chance to interact with the investigating agency and the available close relatives or friends. A sympathetic talk with the relatives not only builds a bond of confidence and faith on the postmortem conducting medical practitioner and forensic medicine but also supply important information about deceased. An autopsy conducting officer must not forget that he is a doctor.

It is advisable that the dead body must be identified by the police personnel in-charge of that dead body and a close relative preferably with good vision and not under the influence of alcohol. The name, age and residential address of the deceased must be verified for their correctness and spellings. This prevents future time consuming complications like informing the officer dealing with notification of deaths, filing insurance forms, property matters etc. The name of the relative and police personnel who identified the body should be mentioned in the autopsy report and they should be informed about the same.

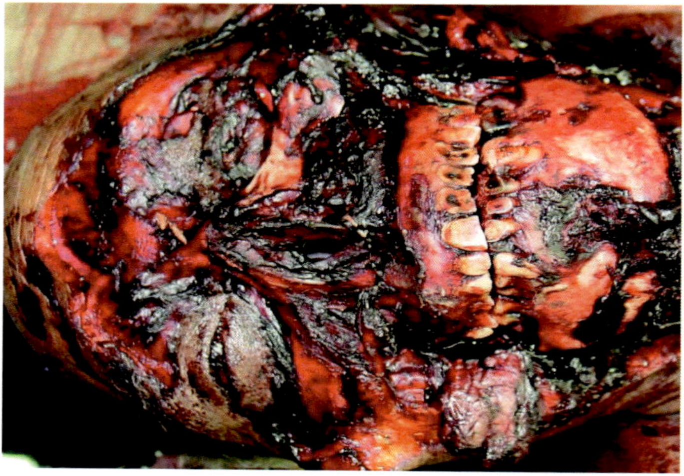

FIGURE 2.1: Difficulties may arise while identifying the decomposed or mutilated dead bodies as in this case (case of face off), where the soft tissue of the face is eaten away by dogs. However clothes, articles and identification marks on the deceased can solve this problem. Note the margin of wound over scalp.

Mentioning as many identification marks as available in the autopsy report (Fig. 2.1) of the unknown deceased is always helpful to the investigating agency to find out relatives of the deceased so that the body can be handed over to the mourners and the last ritual be performed according to the religion of the deceased or his wishes.

TATTOO (FIGS 2.2 TO 2.6)

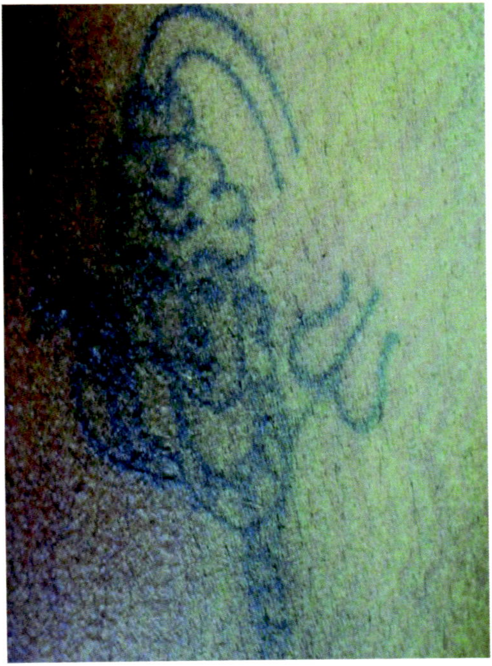

FIGURE 2.2: Tattoo is one of the best identification marks. This tattoo indicates religious belief, god of worship as well as geographic origin of the deceased.

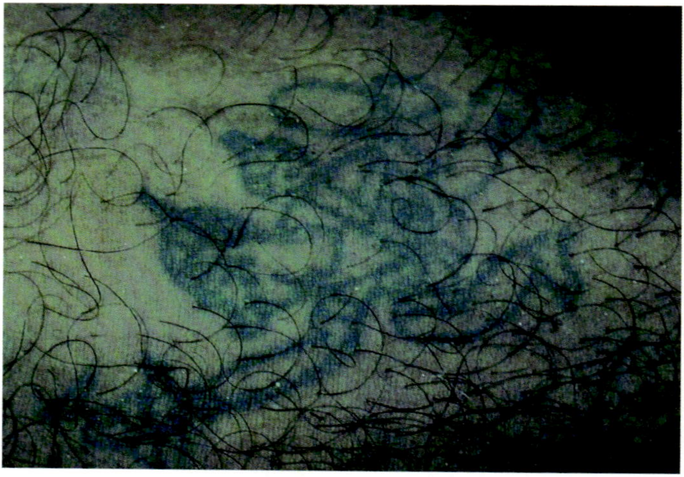

FIGURE 2.3: A tattoo depicting the picture of God Hanuman. The tattoo of God Hanuman will be found only on the body of the male and never on female.

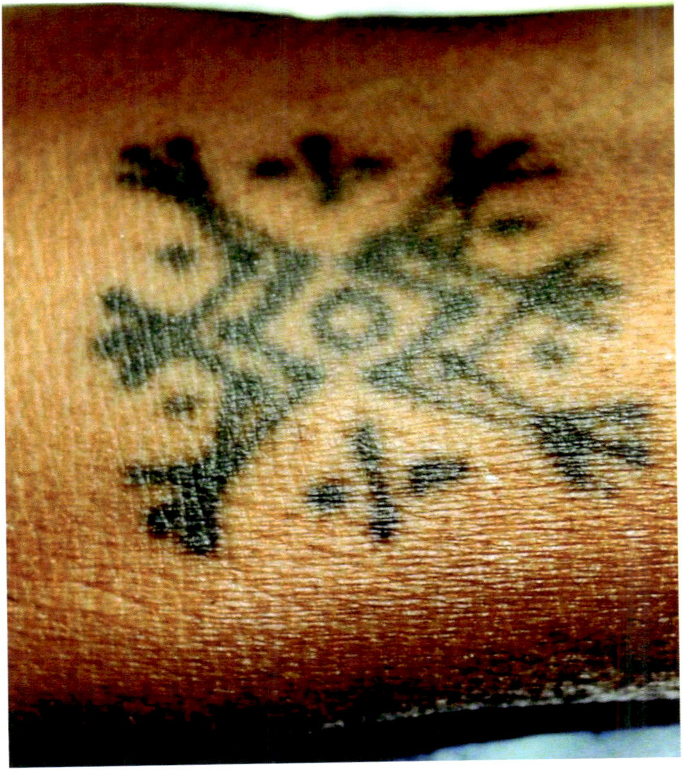

FIGURE 2.4: This tattooed design is a design of crab. This design is tattooed only by females of some tribes in India. As per the tribal belief crab is the most fertile creature and tattooing its design on the body imparts fertility to the tattooed female.

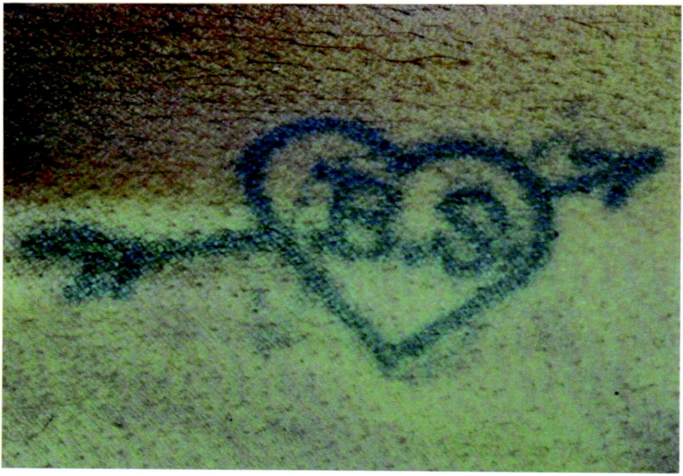

FIGURE 2.5: Some tattoos give or indicate name of the deceased or his beloved or close relative. The language tattooed may indicate the language of the deceased and his educational standard.

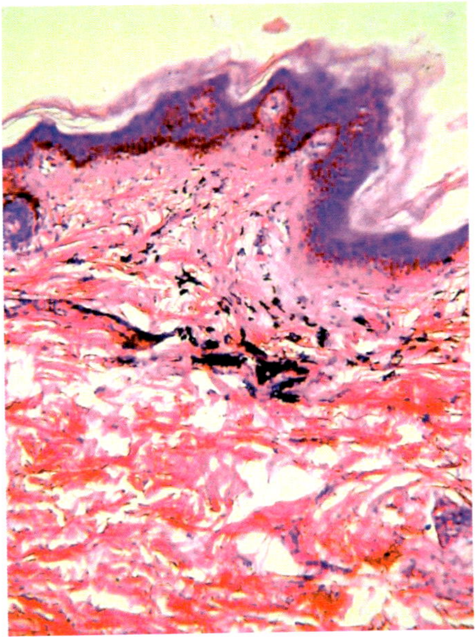

FIGURE 2.6: The advantage of tattoo is that it is not destroyed even after desquamation of skin due to decomposition or in saponification or mummification as the pigments of tattooing material are deposited in the dermis (X100 H and E stain).

SCAR (FIGS 2.7 AND 2.8)

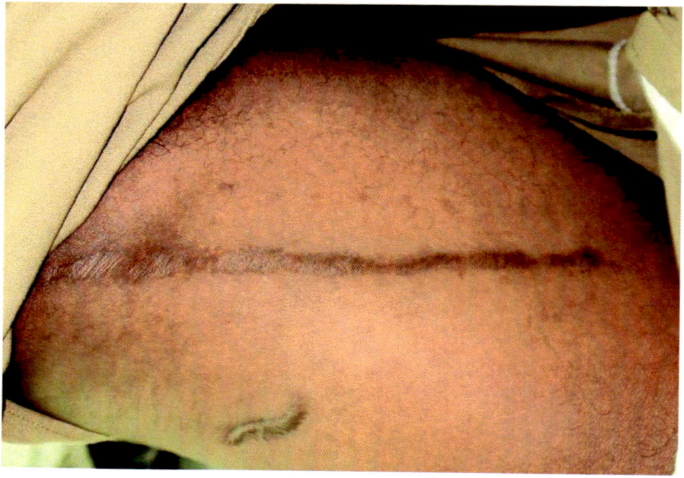

FIGURE 2.7: The second most reliable identification mark is scar. The scar of previous surgery or a peculiar injury is always important as history of surgery or injury is always known to the close relatives.

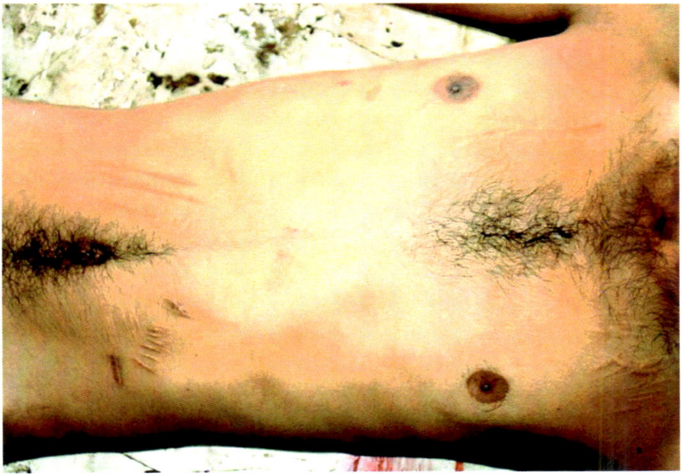

FIGURE 2.8: These are the scars of self inflicted injuries. They indicate previous attempts of suicide.

BIRTH MARKS AND DEFORMITIES (FIGS 2.9 TO 2.11)

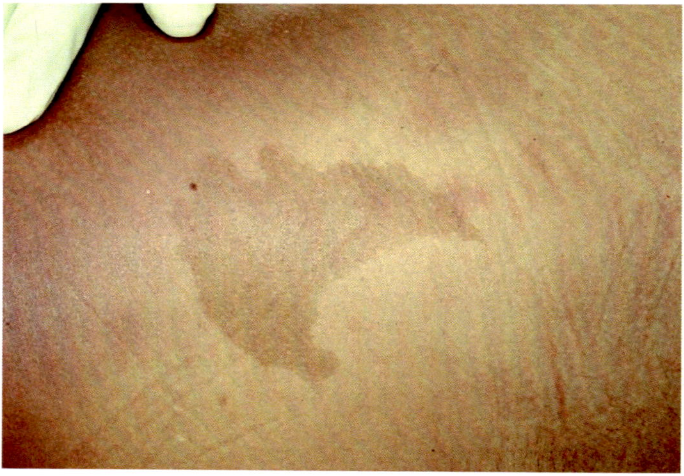

FIGURE 2.9: Birth marks are another peculiar identification marks.

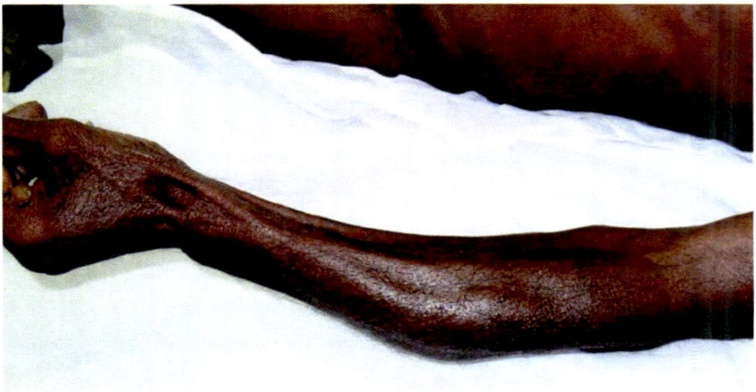

FIGURE 2.10: Old deformities have to be notified in autopsy report as they give clue to the identity of the deceased.

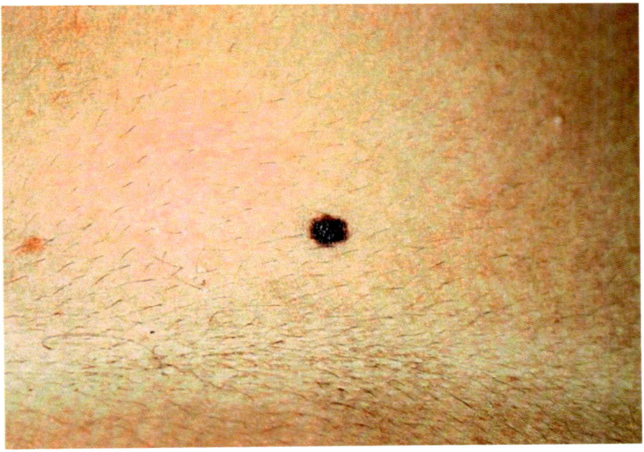

FIGURE 2.11: Moles are good identification marks if they are present on some peculiar sites.

OTHER IDENTIFICATION POINTS (FIGS 2.12 AND 2.13)

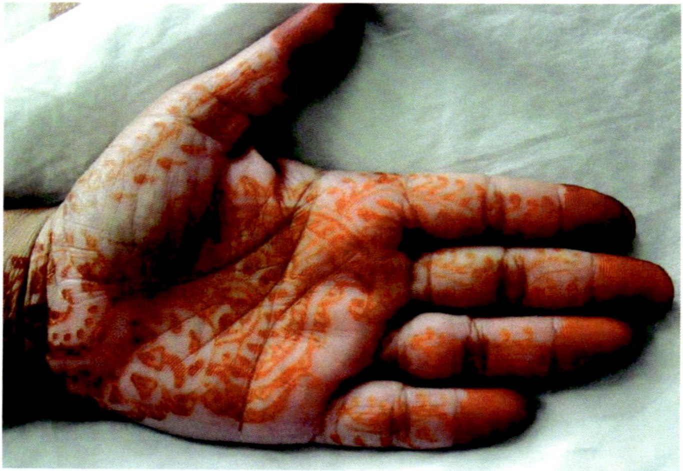

FIGURE 2.12: Certain temporary body staining can be found very useful in identifying a deceased person, e.g. Mehendi stains on palm indicate involvement of deceased in some ceremony in recent past. These stains are visible even on the de-gloved skin due to decomposition.

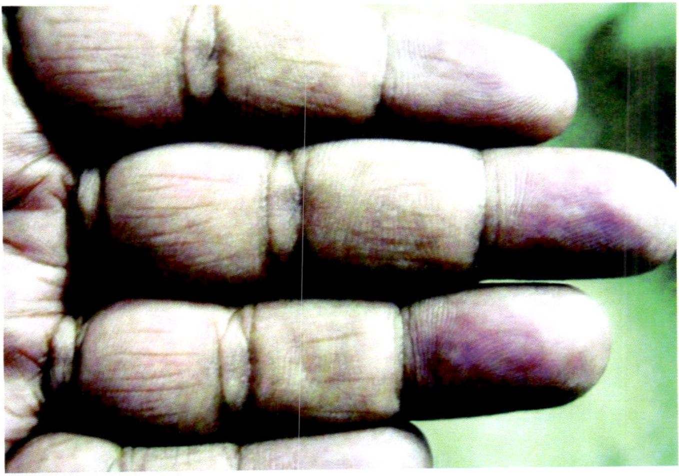

FIGURE 2.13: Finger prints can be collected from the non-decomposed bodies. Hence it should be advised to the investigating agency rather than removing skin from the fingers for this purpose. However when the body is decomposed and skin of palm is present then it can be removed for fingerprinting on demand by investigating agency.

Material from the deceased for blood grouping and DNA profiling can be collected on demand by investigating agency.

In the process of exhumation, the place of burial from where the body is supposed to be exhumed should be identified by as many relatives as present at the time of burial. Their names must be mentioned in the autopsy report.

3 Cloths, Articles and Body Surface

Meticulous examination of articles, cloths and body surface gives clue of contact of the deceased with external objects, atmosphere and much more.

EXAMINATION OF CLOTHES (FIGS 3.1 TO 3.9)

Clothes of the deceased must be examined with respect to damages occurred (cuts, tears, broken buttons, torn button holes, open stitch lines, scorching, burns, etc.), stains (mud, semen, urine, feces, blood, saliva, ink, paint, decomposition fluid, poisons, etc.), foreign bodies (hair, fiber, earth particles, glass particles, etc.), peculiar smell or any other peculiarity.

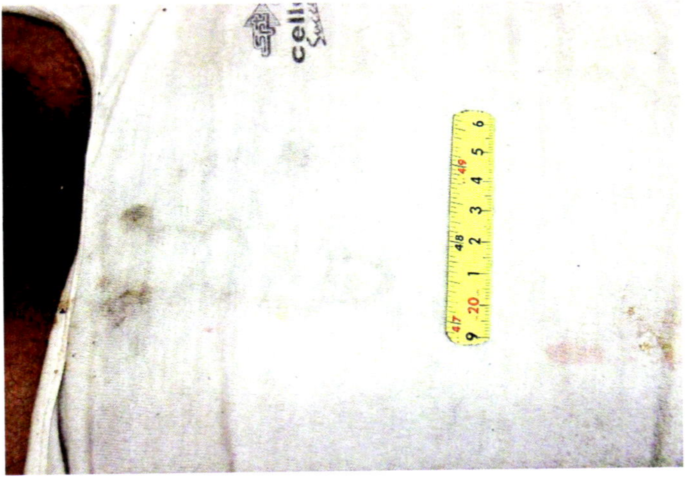

FIGURE 3.1: Saliva stain in cases of hanging is a very important finding. Saliva may trickle down on the clothes over anterior trunk to form a hard to soft saliva stain. These stains may be lost or unnoticeable if condensation occurs on the body which was kept in cold storage and clothes become moist.

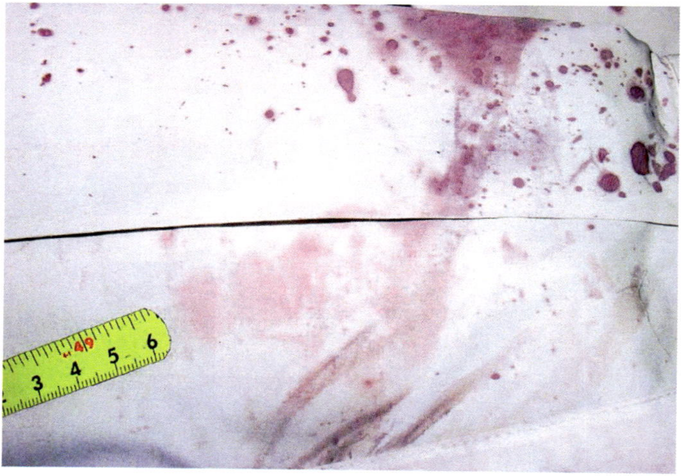

FIGURE 3.2: Blood stains on the clothes give important information like quantity of hemorrhage (cloths are soaked in blood), source of blood, age of stain, etc.

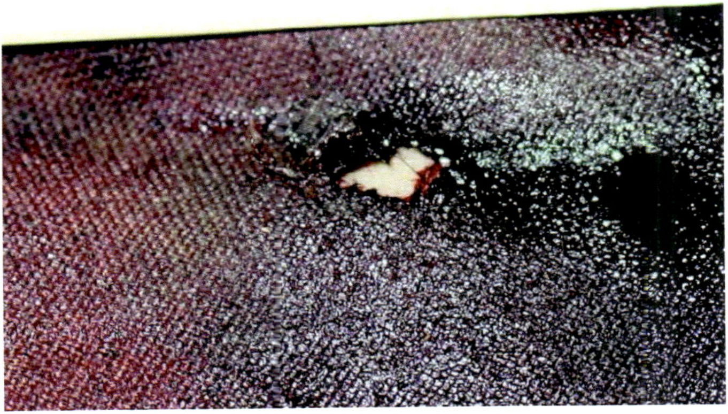

FIGURE 3.3: Examination of the clothes in cases of firearm injuries may show a rent by missile with scorching, blackening or soiling around it, which is essential to determine the range of firing and differentiating entry and exit wound.

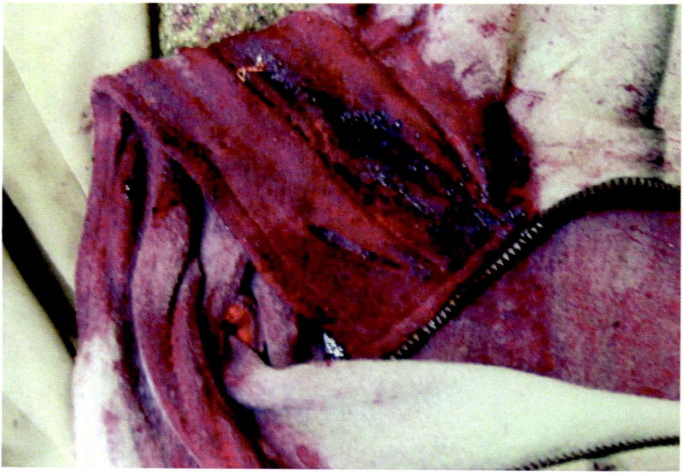

FIGURE 3.4: Cuts on the particular area of the cloth indicate the intention of the assailant. As in this case multiple cuts on the collar indicate the intention of assailant to cut victims throat. Similarly cuts found in the perineal region of trousers or underpants indicate that the assailant had intention to injure or mutilate genitalia.

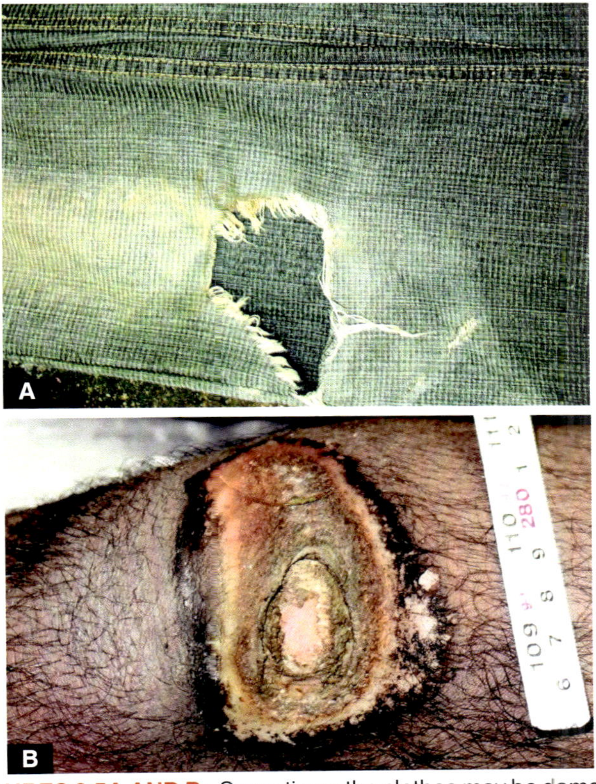

FIGURES 3.5A AND B: Some times the clothes may be damaged after death of the person wearing them. In this case the damage is caused due to friction of the clothes and subjacent body part of the flowing body to the wall of water canal.

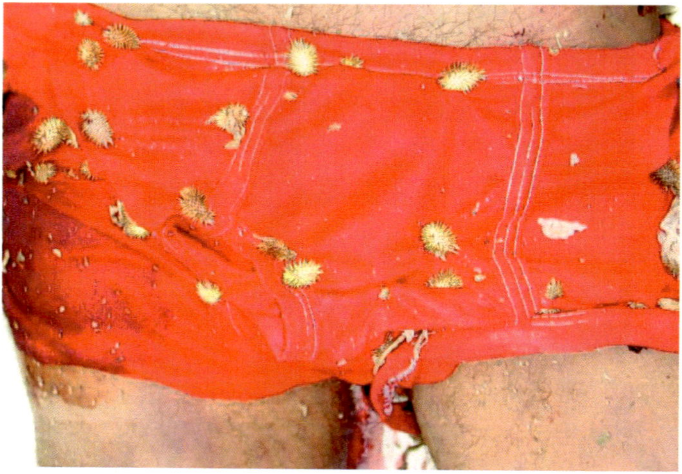

FIGURE 3.6: Foreign bodies are important trace evidences to prove contacts. In this case the spiny dried burlike fruits (locally called as Gokhru) attached at places to the underpants indicates that the body must be lying in bushes without any trousers.

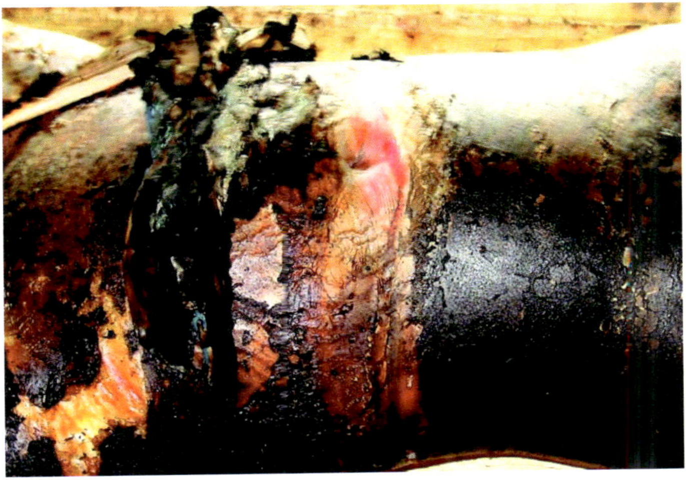

FIGURE 3.7: Examination of clothes in cases of burns and scalds can give information like smell of inflammable substance used. They must be preserved for detection of inflammable substance even if there is no peculiar odor.

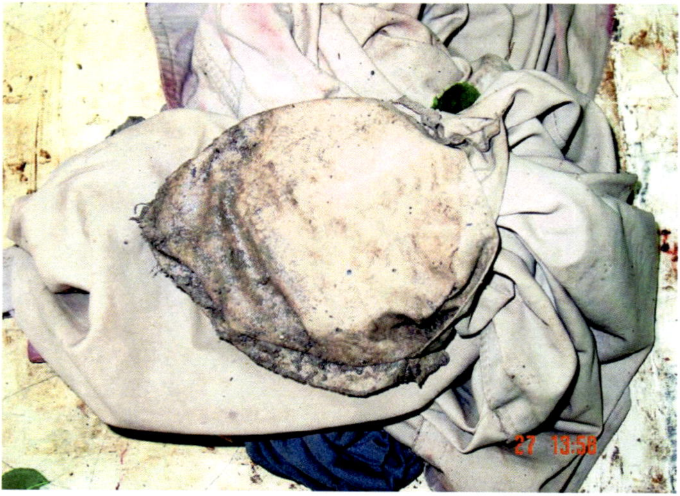

FIGURE 3.8: Examination of pockets of cloths give valuable information, e.g. traces of tobacco, ganja or cocaine may be found if the deceased was in a habit of consuming the same or dealt in its trade. In this case mud was found in the pockets of a drowned victim proving contact with the water.

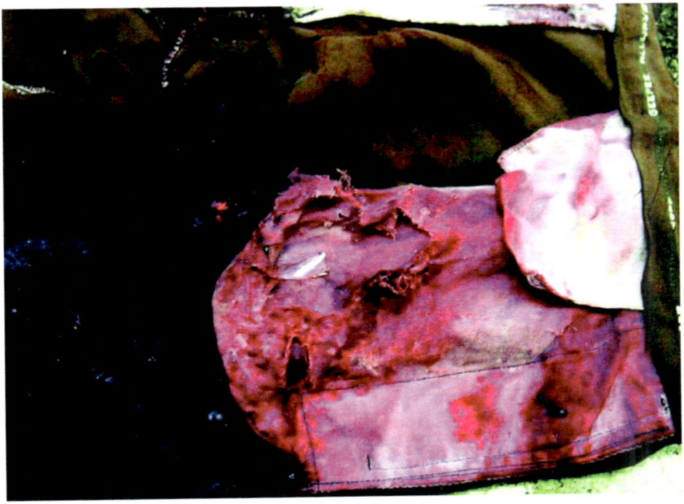

FIGURE 3.9: A photograph of the pocket of trousers. The drunkard victim died in a vehicular accident with a bottle of liquor in his pocket. The bottle broke into pieces and caused injuries to scrotum and subjacent thigh region.

EXAMINATION OF ARTICLES ON THE BODY (FIGS 3.10 TO 3.12)

Damage to articles on the body like ornaments, spectacles, coins or keys is also important piece of information, e.g. arcing, melting, deformation or magnetization of metal articles is very important finding to suggest damages caused by lightning.

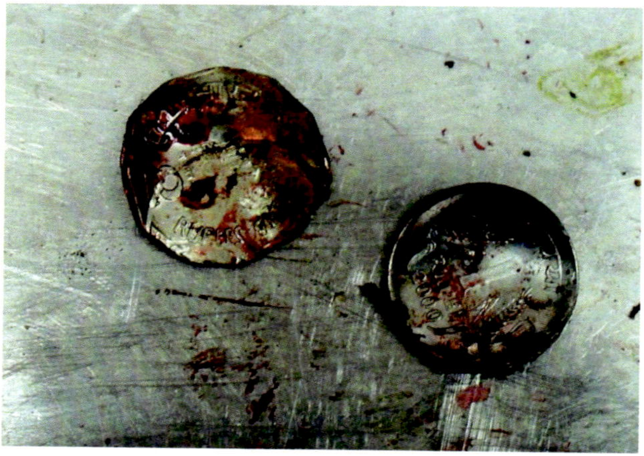

FIGURE 3.10: These are the coins in the pocket of trousers of a victim who was crushed by train over railway track.

Other articles like weapon or part of weapon found in or outside the body should be removed properly; air dried without washing and packed in a paper bag and plastic bag with few small rents for breathing of biological articles and avoiding decomposition.

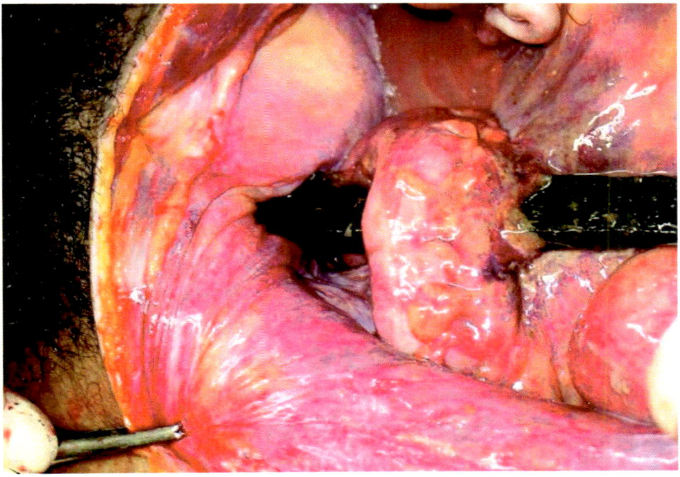

FIGURE 3.11: A part of wooden plank from fence which was impaled in the abdomen through anus. A part of impaled wooden plank was removed before death in casualty department. Rest of the part remained in abdomen and was removed at autopsy.

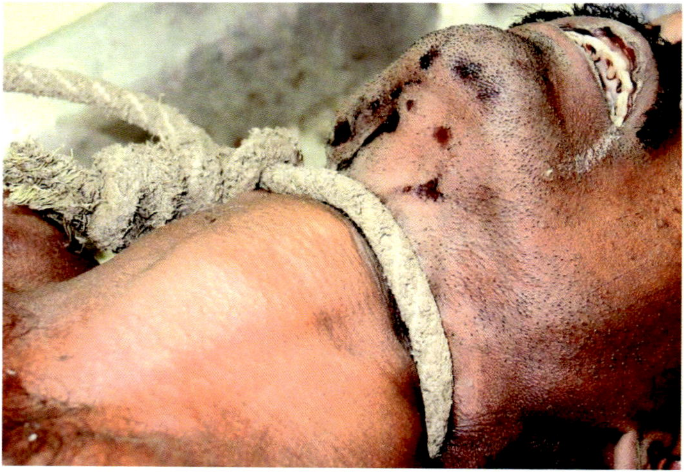

FIGURE 3.12: Ligature material tied around neck, wrists, arms and legs must be examined carefully for its strength, texture, color, thickness, length of loop or noose and free end, types and numbers of knots or any other peculiarity. It should be removed by cutting opposite to the knot so that the knots can be preserved.

EXAMINATION OF BODY SURFACE (FIGS 3.13 TO 3.19)

The body surface of the deceased should be examined for foreign bodies, stains and damages. If the killer is a woman or is weaker than the victim, then chili powder may be found on face, neck and in the eyes of the deceased.

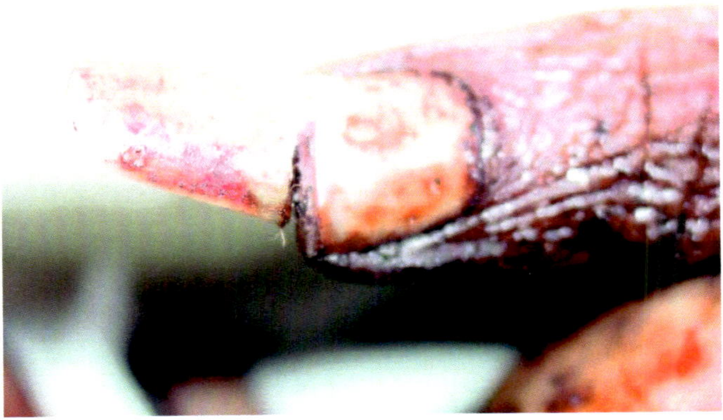

FIGURE 3.13: Nails should be examined in all cases of homicide and sexual offence for their damages and the material under the nails. Nail clippings should be collected in all cases of homicide for biological examination by forensic science laboratory. Note the fabric fibers entangled in the broken nail. They should be sent along with clothes of victim and that of suspected accused to forensic science lab for comparison. Victim's clothes should be used as control sample.

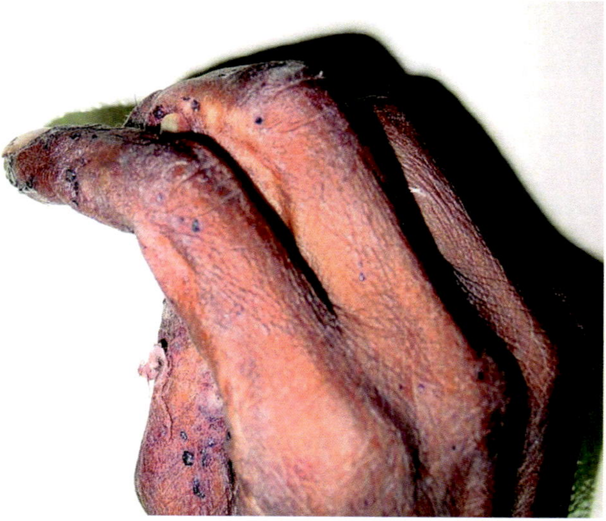

FIGURE 3.14: Foreign hair or hairs may be found in hand or on other body parts like female breast or genitalia. This hair along with hair and blood of suspected accused and that of victim as a control sample should be sent for biological study by forensic science lab.

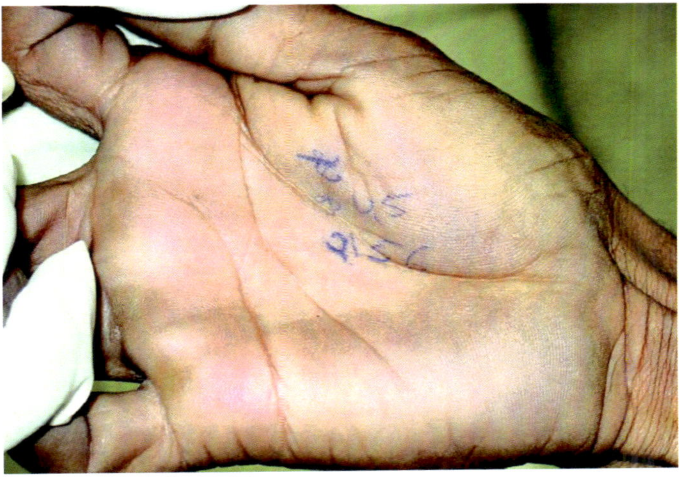

FIGURE 3.15: Examination of palm may reveal an important information as some persons have habit of taking notes on palm, e.g. phone numbers, addresses, reminders or calculating or they test ball pen by writing or lining on palm. Some people even write suicidal notes on their palm.

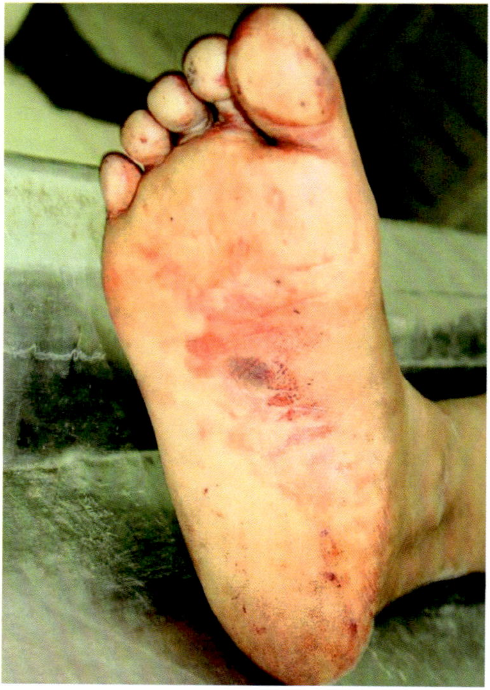

FIGURE 3.16: Examination of soles of feet may show mud stains, blood stains, etc. This photograph shows blood stains on the sole of a lady, died due to postpartum hemorrhage.

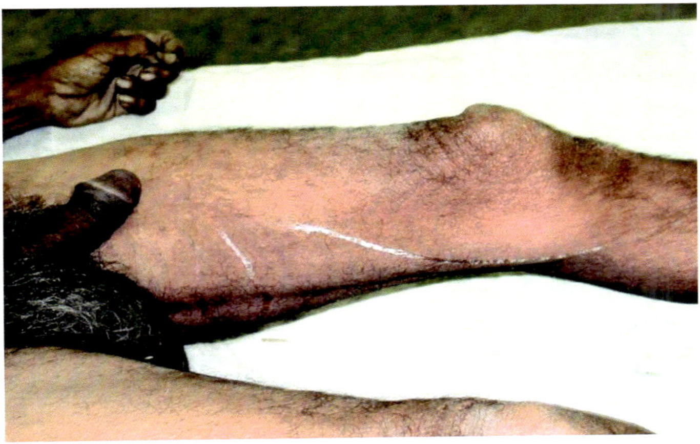

FIGURE 3.17: Purging of semen in a case of partial hanging. Note the dried trickled semen indicating the posture of the deceased till drying of the stain. These type of stains can be lost if condensation occurs on the dead body removed from cold storage.

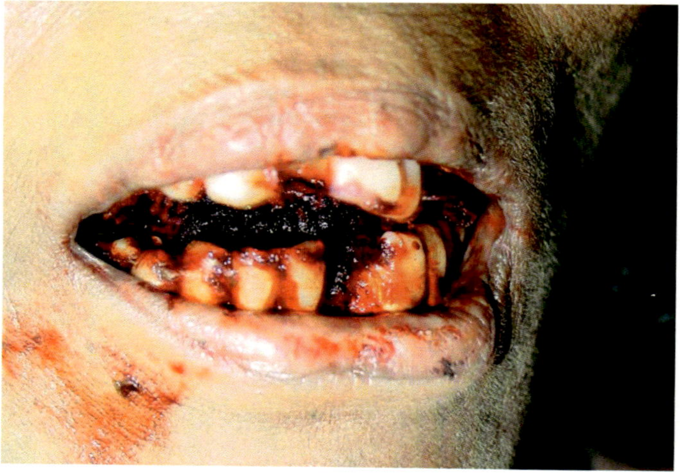

FIGURE 3.18: Examination of nostrils, ears, eyes, buccal cavity and teeth is an important area of examination and must be examined in each autopsy. Presence of tobacco under lower lip, chewable leaf (Pan) or gutka in oral cavity are commonly found in unnatural deaths.

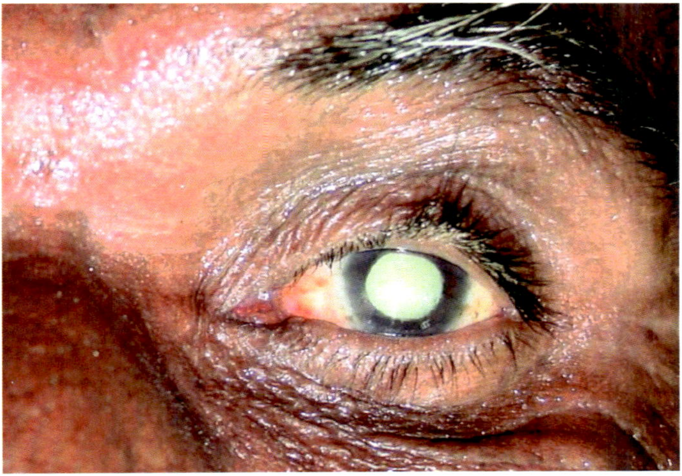

FIGURE 3.19: Examination of eyes of the non-decomposed body under good light can also reveal findings like cataract.

4 Changes After Death

Knowledge of changes after death is very much essential to determine the time since death and accuracy of interpretation of injuries. Following death the changes depends on intrinsic factors like physical health of body, disease, infection or injury by which the victim died, sex and age of deceased, body temperature at the time of death, etc. and extrinsic factors like clothing, atmospheric temperature, humidity, media in which the body kept, air currents etc. Hence all the factors must be considered to evaluate time since death. Now, many mortuaries have cold storage to preserve dead bodies. However they create difficulties in calculating time since death as their low temperature delays the changes occurring in the dead body.

EARLY CHANGES AFTER DEATH (FIGS 4.1 TO 4.3)

A death certifying doctor usually comes across these changes. They can be enumerated as permanent cessation of circulation and respiration, skin becomes pale and dry, muscles become flaccid and there is absence of corneal and papillary reflex. The temperature of body decreases with passing time.

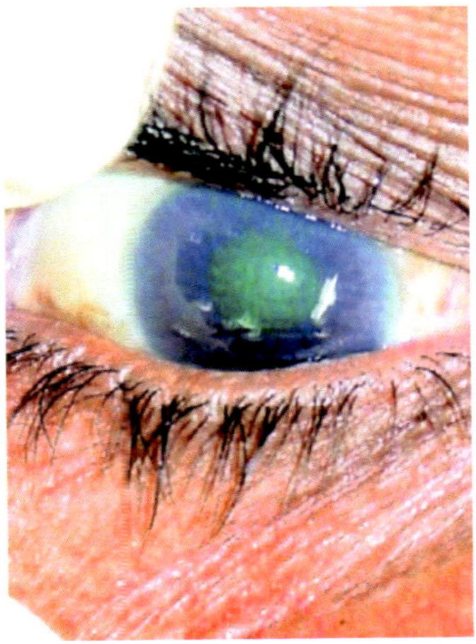

FIGURE 4.1: Haziness of cornea can be detected as early as seven minutes after death. It depends on the dryness of atmospheric air as well as whether the eyelids were closed or open. For ophthalmoscopy after death this haziness can be removed by cleaning the cornea for about one to two minutes with normal saline.

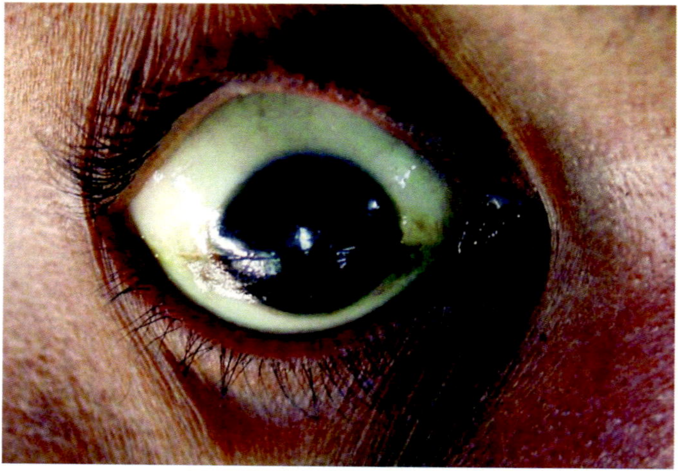

FIGURE 4.2: By passing time if the eyelids remain partially open or open then the dust and dirt settles on the sclera and cornea called as tache noire.

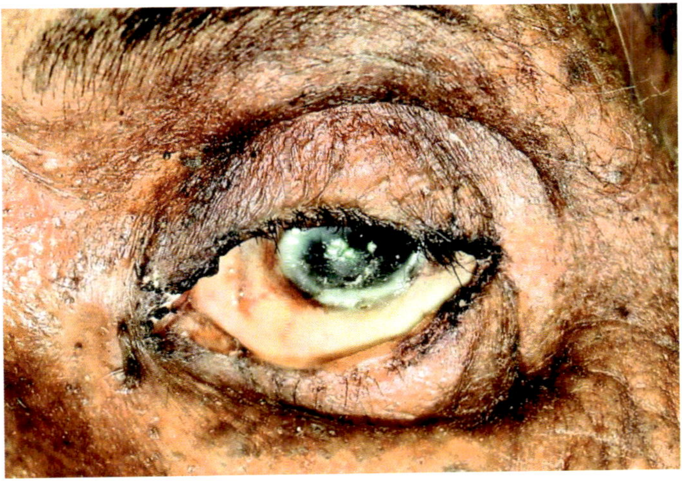

FIGURE 4.3: Intraocular tension decreases following death and the eyeballs become grossly flabby after about 6 to 7 hours and can be noticed earlier in e derly persons.

LATE CHANGES AFTER DEATH (FIGS 4.4 TO 4.30)

The medical practitioner conducting autopsy may come across these changes if the autopsy of the deceased is conducted after some time of death.

Although pallor and contact flattening of the dead body can be noticed immediately following death, it can be truly appreciated after appearance of postmortem lividity.

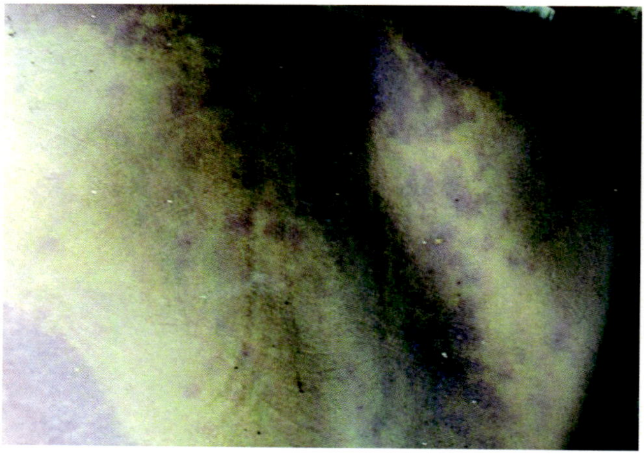

FIGURE 4.4: The postmortem lividity starts appearing in the dependent part of the dead body and is noticeable in about half an hour following death in a fair person. First it appears in patches in dependent uncompressed part. However its appreciation depends on the quantity of blood in the body and complexion of the deceased.

FIGURE 4.5: The patches of postmortem lividity coalesce and become darker in six to eight hours. However the lividity can be displaced by compressing the area of lividity for about five minutes. When it is not fixed.

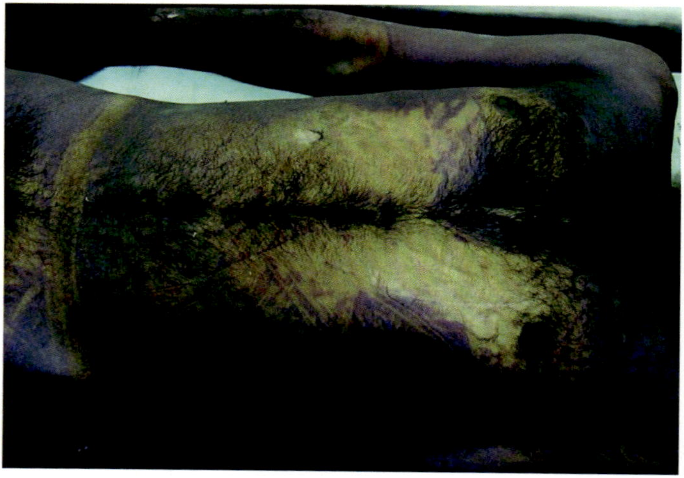

FIGURE 4.6: The postmortem lividity becomes fixed in about ten to fourteen hours. Postmortem lividity can give valuable information like, time since death, position of body after death, changes in the position after death and probable cause of death.

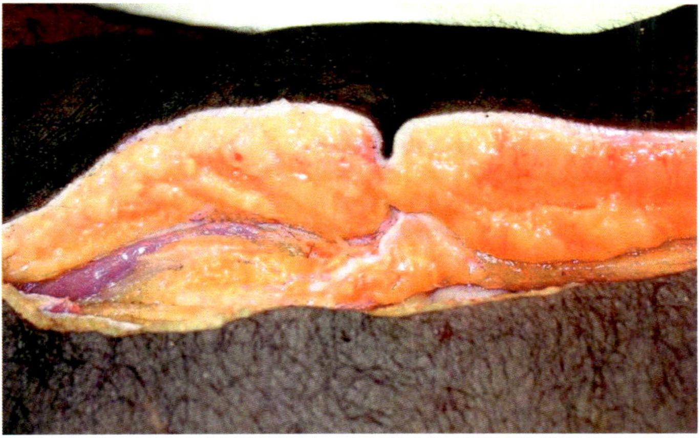

FIGURE 4.7: Cut section in the region of fixed post-mortem lividity. Note the subcutaneous and fat tissue. Compare this photograph with Figure 5.2, i.e. contusion.

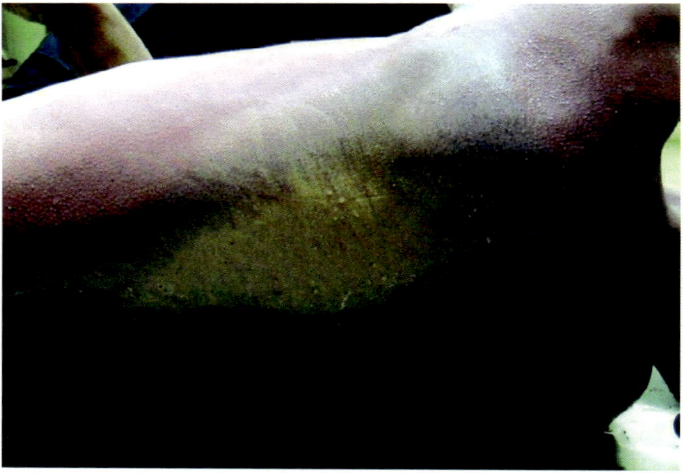

FIGURE 4.8: Sometimes different shades of postmortem lividity may be seen in the same dead body. This dead body was kept between ice slabs overnight for preservation purpose.

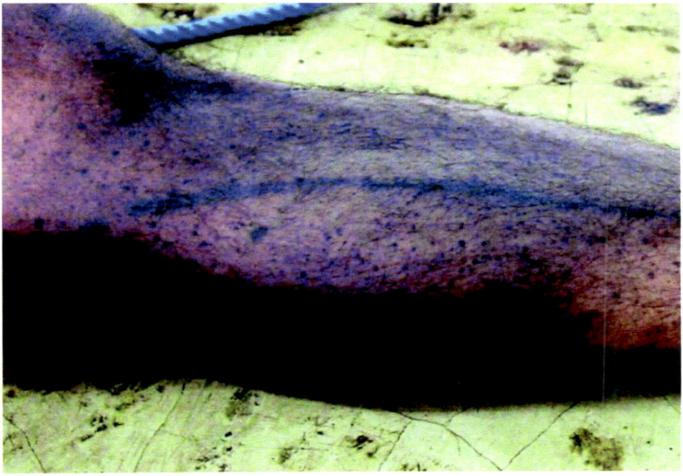

FIGURE 4.9: Many times petechial hemorrhages can be noticed in the postmortem lividity. It's a postmortem phenomenon and should not be mistaken for any cause of death.

The postmortem lividity disappears with commencement of decomposition.

With postmortem lividity another two changes after death can be noticeable. The first one is progressive cooling of body and other is body stiffening, i.e. rigor mortis. Temperature of the body can be noticed at many sites, e.g. deep rectal, ear, deep nasal, etc. Rigor mortis can be felt by flexing or extending the joints. Always suspecting that the rigor might have been broken by relatives or people who handled the body before autopsy is helpful in its evaluation. Rigor mortis disappear with autolytic changes in the muscles.

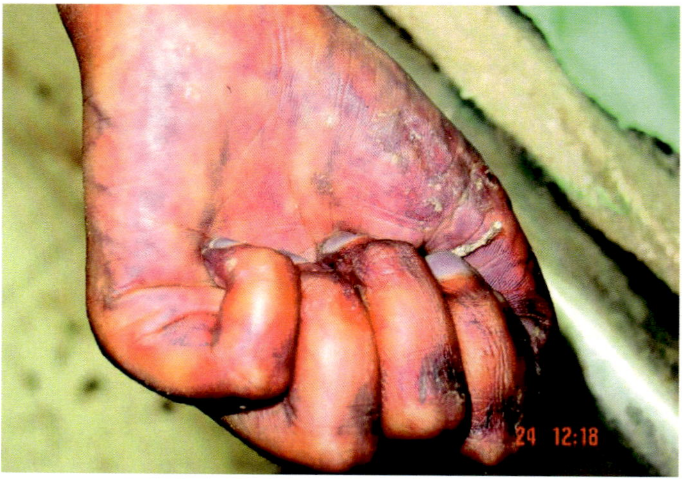

FIGURE 4.10: Instantaneous rigor or cadaveric spasm can be noticed in death due to drowning, suicidal firearm injury, etc. It is considered as a last act of a dying victim. It is usually noticed as firm grasped material or weapon in hand.

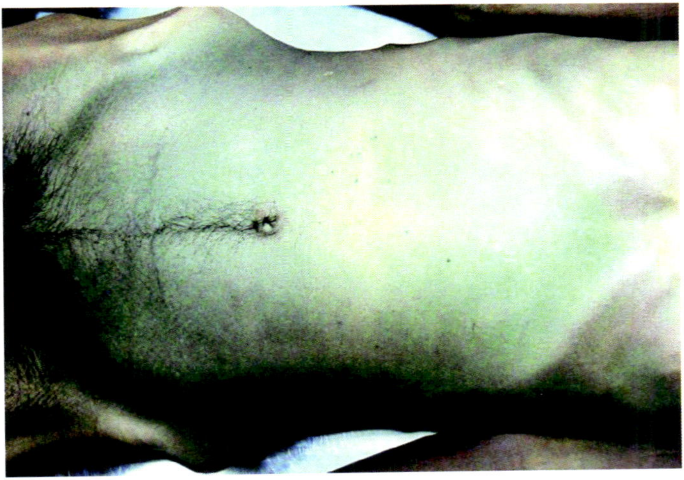

FIGURE 4.11: The first external sign of decomposition is greenish discoloration of anterior abdominal wall when the body is lying through out period on back, after death.

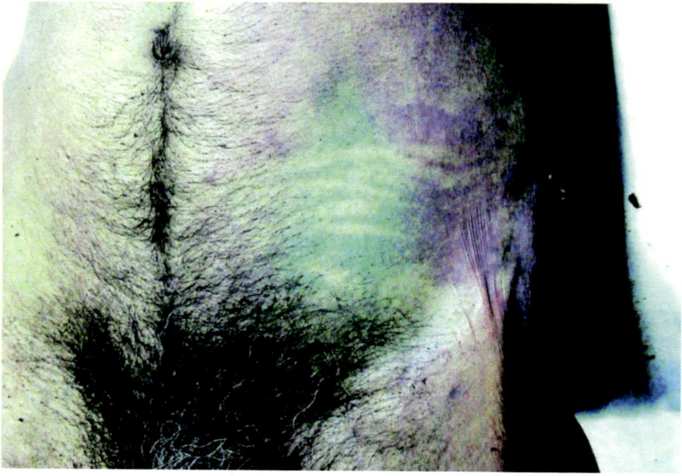

FIGURE 4.12: If the body is lying on abdomen after death, the postmortem lividity developed in that region may acquire greenish discoloration rather than the area of skin of that region where the lividity is not developed. This finding may be found in a nondecomposed body and should not be considered as a sign of decomposition. Compare this figure with Figure 4.11 where skin of the abdomen is discolored whereas in this figure it is only area of postmortem lividity and not the skin.

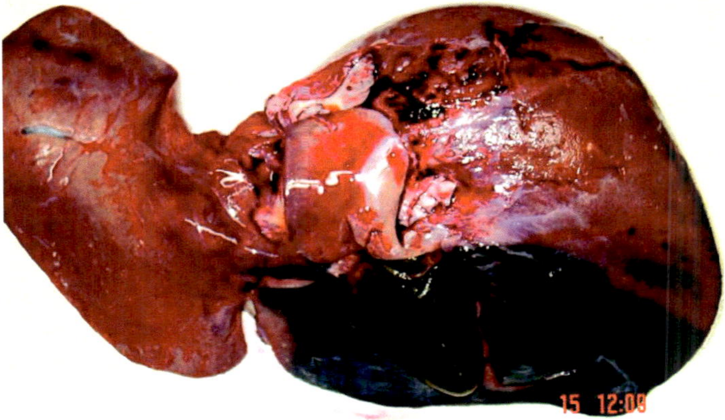

FIGURE 4.13: The first internal sign of decomposition is greenish discoloration of undersurface of liver which can be noticed after twelve to fourteen hours after death. This discoloration occurs due to contact with subjacent transverse colon.

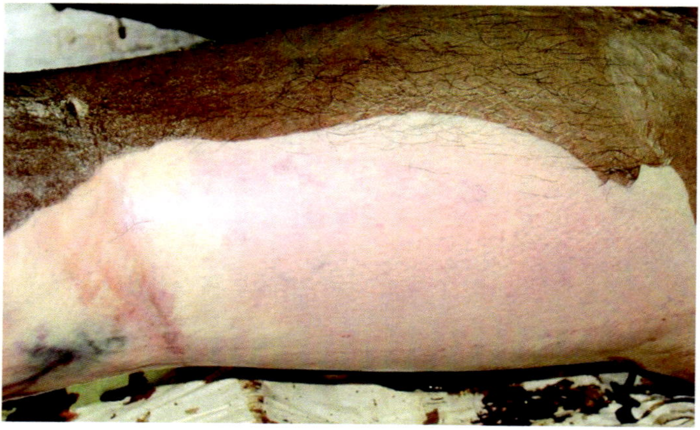

FIGURE 4.14: Desquamation of skin occurs early in summer. It may also be seen over most handled part of the dead body.

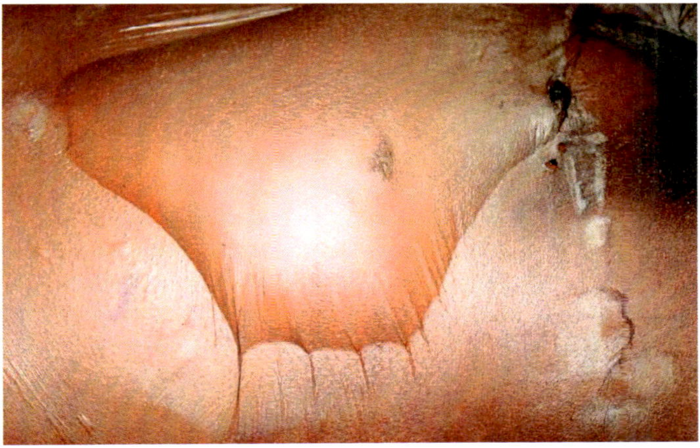

FIGURE 4.15: Presence of bullae containing foul smelling gases and very little amount of reddish watery foul smelling non proteineous fluid is one of the early signs of decomposition.

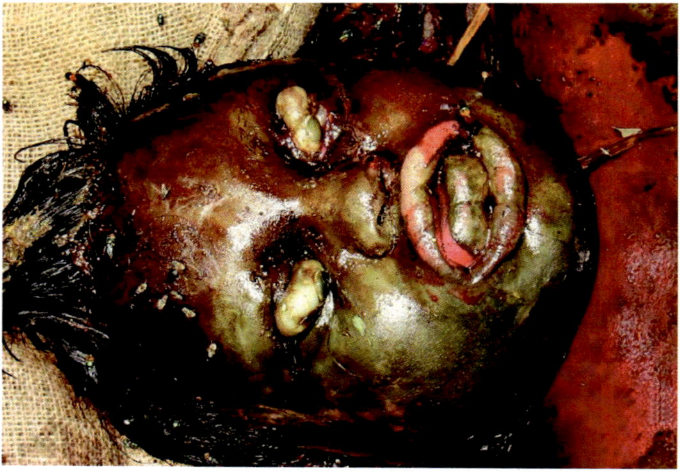

FIGURE 4.16A: The gases collect in the tissue so that complete body swells. Gross crepitations can be felt on compression of body parts. Reddish watery foul smelling fluid starts oozing with gases from mouth and nostrils. Eyes protruded out with swollen protruded tongue. Hair is easily plucked. Greenish discoloration of body is very obvious at this stage. All these findings amount to gross decomposition. At the rear end feces purge out and rectum and uterine contents in a pregnant deceased may prolapse. Stomach contents also purge out through mouth and nostrils.

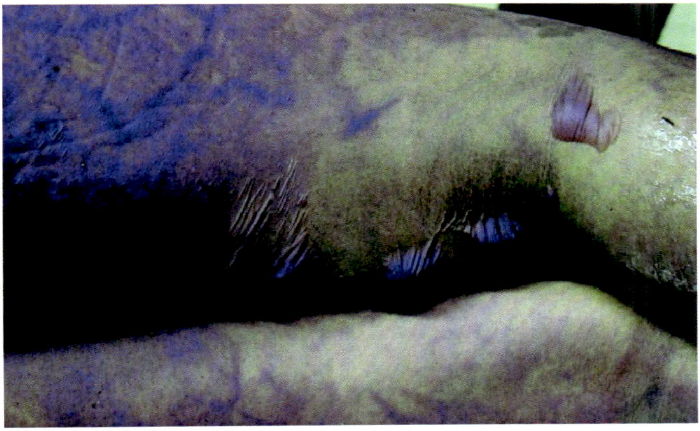

FIGURE 4.16B: With advancing decomposition, reddish watery fluid with small amount of gases started collecting under the epidermis in the dependent part of the body. Compare this photograph with Figure 4.15. The proportion of gases and fluid depends on the factor that on which part the bullae is present. If it is present on the dependent part of the body, it contains more quantity of darker fluid than that of gases and if it is present on non-dependent part of the body then it contains more amounts of gases than light colored fluid. These changes can be mistaken as burn injury.

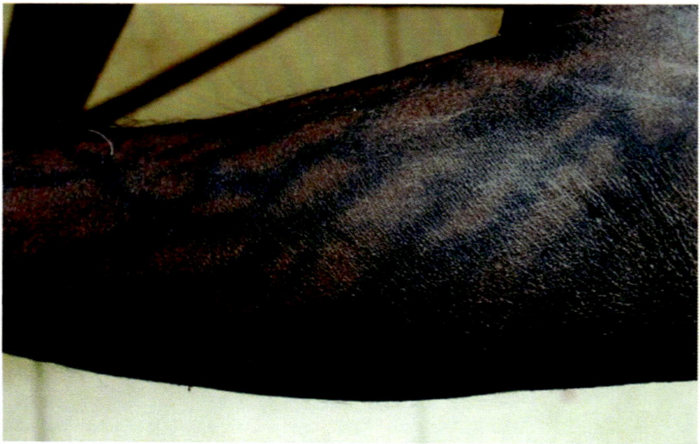

FIGURE 4.17: One gross sign of decomposition is marbling.

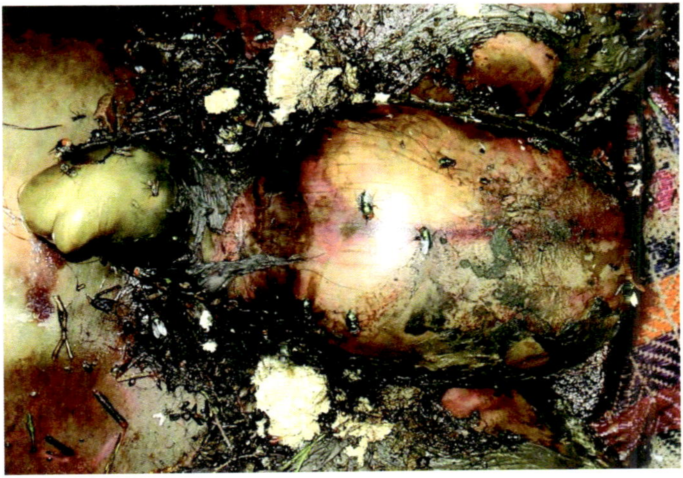

FIGURE 4.18: At this stage of decomposition the fly attract towards the corpse and lay their eggs as white clusters.

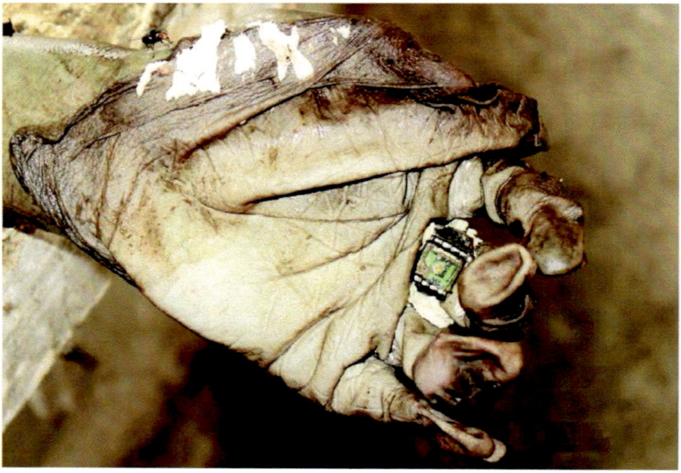

FIGURE 4.19: The complete skin of the hand can be easily removed which is known as degloving.

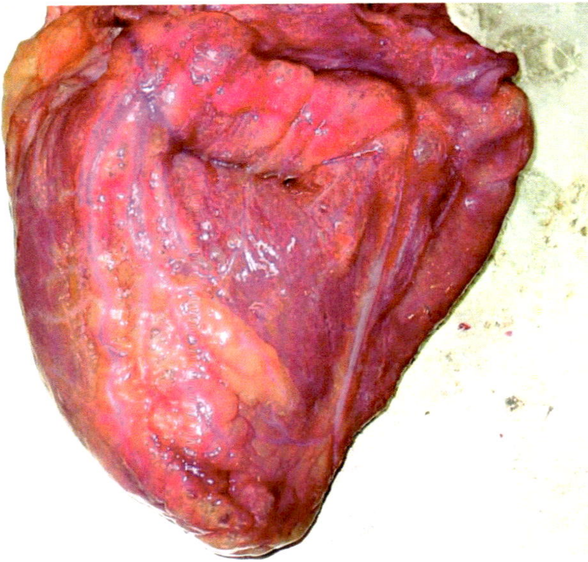

FIGURE 4.20: Internally the organs become either pink, faint pink or dark brown; gases are present in the organ tissue and they are flabby however recognizable in early stages of decomposition. But later on it converts into fragile foul smelling mass. Old myocardial infarcts and atherosclerotic changes are preserved even in advanced decomposition.

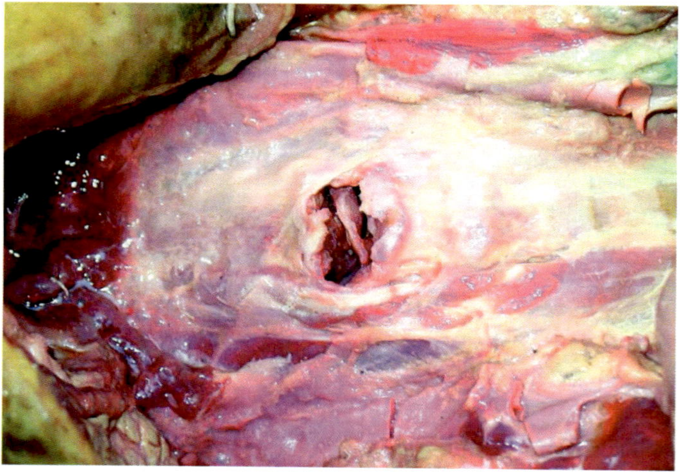

FIGURE 4.21: In advanced stage of decomposition the cartilages and vertebral disk starts shrinking. It may be misinterpreted as fractures and dislocation.

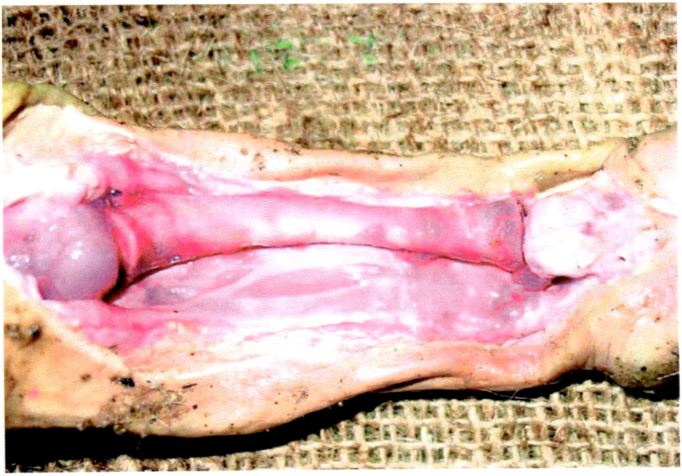

FIGURE 4.22: The developing ends of long bones of the fetus separate from shaft in gross decomposition.

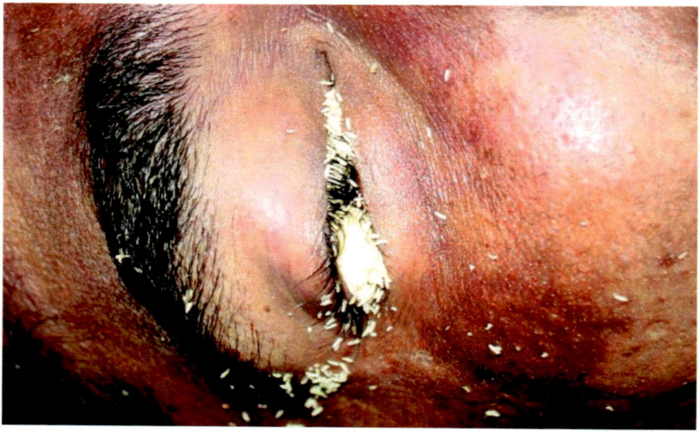

FIGURE 4.23: Infestation of the fly may occur even before the decomposition if the environmental conditions are favorable to them. In this case the maggots were present under the eyelids without any sign of decomposition in the body.

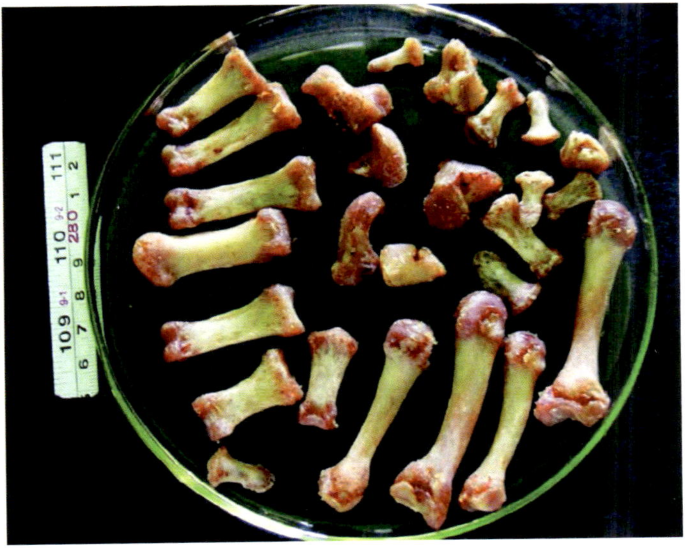

FIGURE 4.24: With passing time the body gets skeletonized. The fresh bones are moist, greasy, tags of tendons may be present, they emit a peculiar smell and periostium may still be present. Time taken for skeletonization depends on where the body is lying. It occurs early when the body is on the ground while delayed when the body is buried.

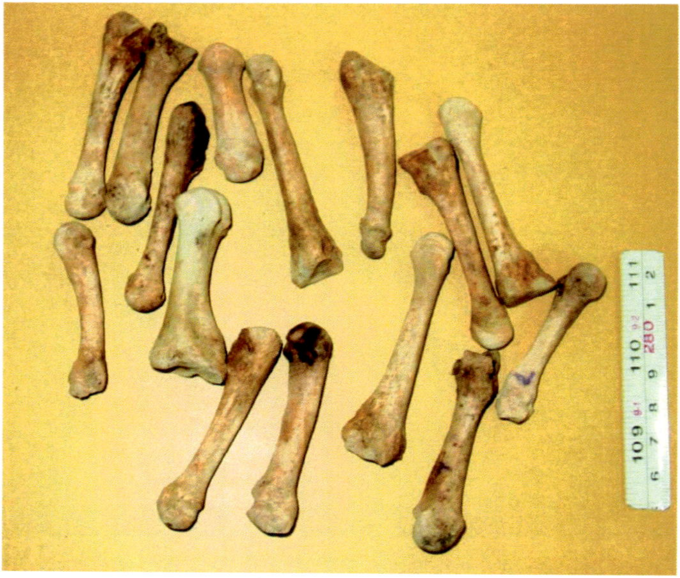

FIGURE 4.25: These are the bones of deceased after about ten years. Note they are dry, without any soft tissue, dried areas of fungal growth present at places.

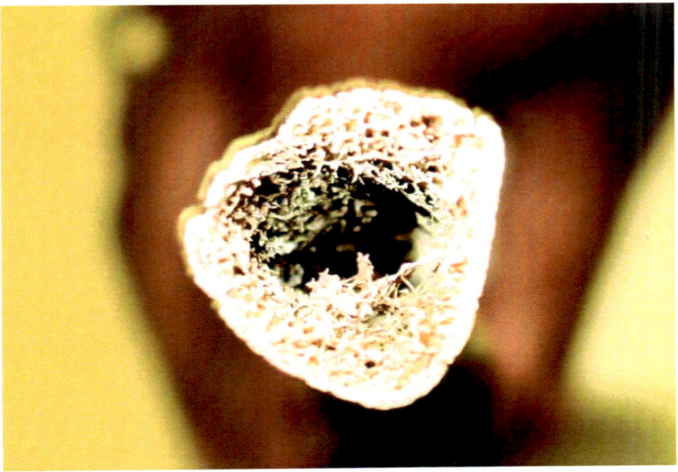

FIGURE 4.26: The cross section of about ten year old bone showing complete loss of organic stroma.

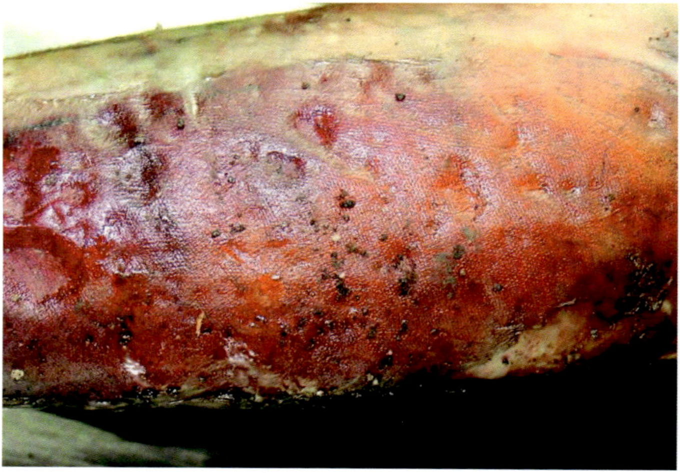

FIGURE 4.27: Sometimes, rather than undergoing colliquative putrifaction followed by skeletonization the process of decomposition modifies and there is adipocere formation. The body parts and surface wounds are preserved in this modification. It may even show the pattern of weaving of the cloth in which the body was wrapped.

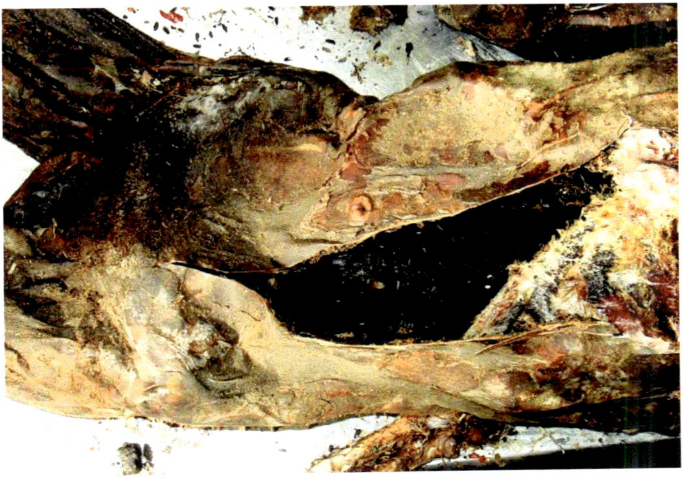

FIGURE 4.28: When the dead body is exposed to dry, airy, hot atmosphere the body can desiccate and become mummified. On opening the abdominal cavity, it can be found that the organs were converted into black thick mass and in late stages it disappeared. Characteristics of surface wounds are preserved.

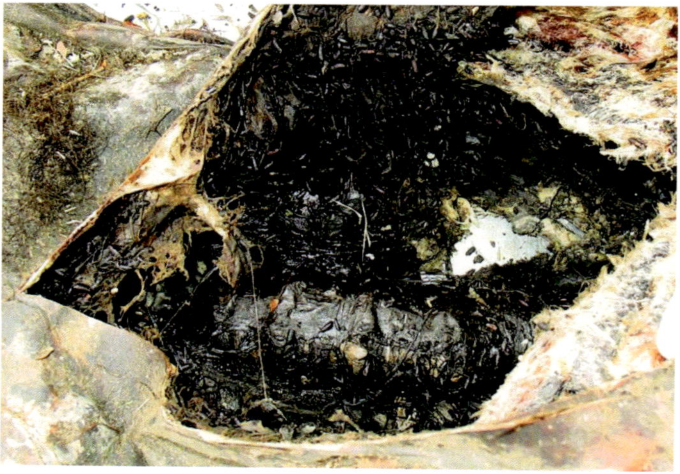

FIGURE 4.29: There were pupae of insect in the abdominal cavity of the mummified body.

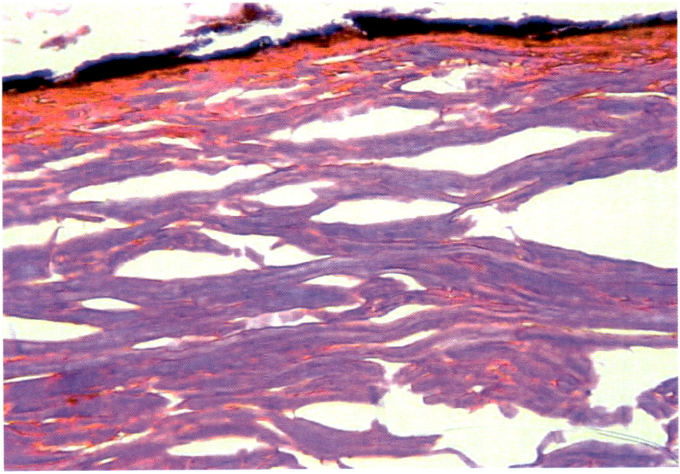

FIGURE 4.30: Note the preserved epidermis and dermis in a mummified body (X100 H and E stain). Antemortem injuries in mummified body are also well preserved and their characteristics are definable on gross and histological study.

Injuries may modify with advancing decomposition, e.g. the red watery fluid starts oozing from non-bleeding wounds.

5 Mechanical Injury

INTRODUCTION—INJURY

Simplest possible definition of injury is 'Breach or breakage in the continuity of the tissue'. There are two types of injuries possible viz. natural and unnatural. Natural injury includes injuries like ulcers, carcinomas, etc. As they don't have any medicolegal significance they are outside the realm of this subject. However it is recommended that the medical practitioner must be able to differentiate between natural injuries and diseases from un-natural injuries.

Un-natural injuries can be further classified according to their causative agent, e.g. when they are caused by force or when physics is involved in their causation or when they are caused by some weapon or object they are mechanical injuries, when they are caused by heat they are burns, etc.

Mechanical Injuries

These are injuries caused by force or mechanics, i.e. physics is involved in causation of these injuries. So their type and severity depend on the type of the weapon, the force applied and the body part struck. Other factors like surface area of the weapon from which the force is transmitted to the body and the body surface area on which the force is transmitted.

INJURIES CAUSED BY BLUNT FORCE (FIGS 5.1 TO 5.28)

Injuries such as bruises or contusions, abrasions and lacerations are caused by the impact of a blunt object on the body part.

Bruises are injuries externally visible where there is no breach in the continuity of skin and they are caused by breakage of small blood vessels causing extravasation of blood in the deeper layers of skin or deeper tissue, most commonly fat tissue.

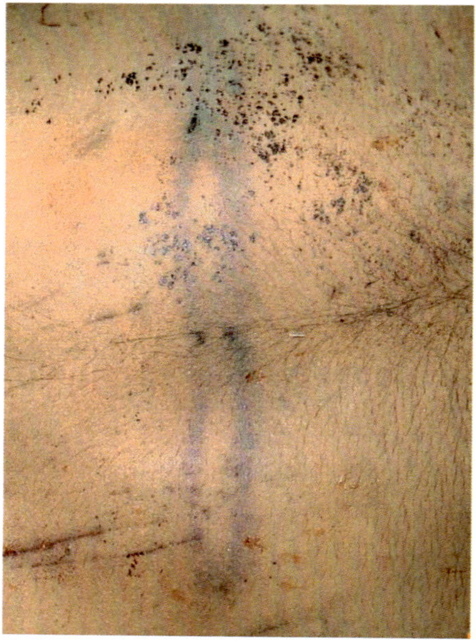

FIGURE 5.1: When they are caused by an object like club or iron rod they depict the imprint of the object and called as tram-line or rail-road bruise.

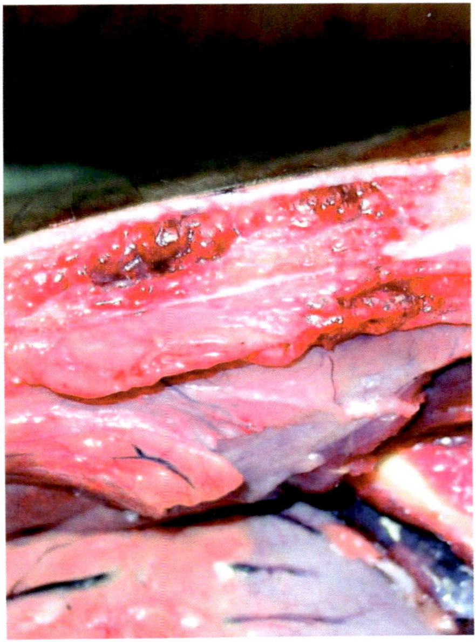

FIGURE 5.2: The advantage of examination of bruise in deceased is that it can be dissected and its extent can be determined. As shown in this figure, the bruise in Figure 5.1 is dissected and found that it is confined to underlying fat and muscle tissue. Although this recent bruise is externally bluish red in color, it is red on internal examination.

Externally visible color of the bruise is considered as a marker for determination of age of the bruise. However there is no clock and calendar for color changes in the bruise to determine its age as the notified color depends on the color recognition ability of the medical practitioner, color of the skin, time since death and the part of body on which it is present, e.g. inability of a medical practitioner to define the exact color of bruise may lead to wrong calculation of age of the bruise, the deceased with dark complexion may not display any color of bruise externally or if it is displayed it looks darker as compared to that of a fair complexioned deceased, with passing time after death the bruise becomes darker, the bruises on the part of body where the postmortem lividity is present are more bluish as compared to those where the postmortem lividity is not present.

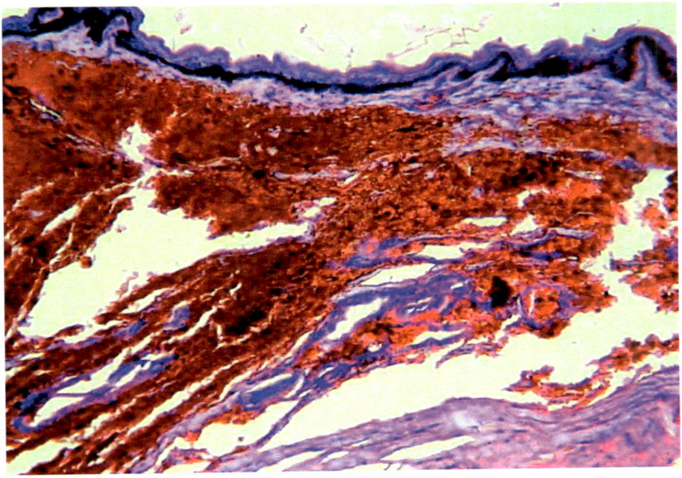

FIGURE 5.3: In superficial bruises the extravasation of blood occurs in the deeper layer of the skin and such bruises are sharply defined on external examination (X100 H and E stain).

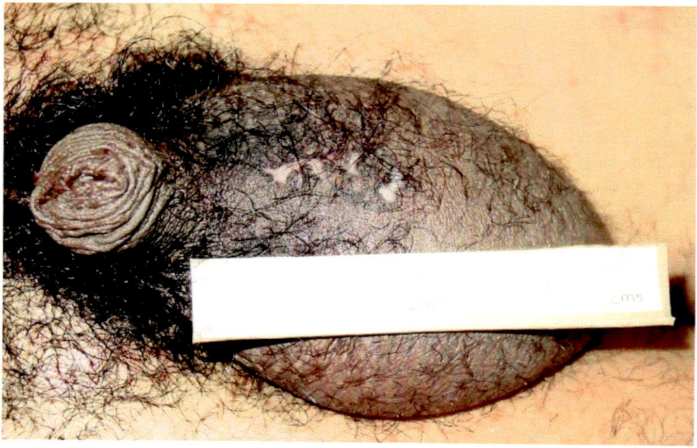

FIGURE 5.4: Complexion of the scrotal skin of an adult is darker as compared to skin of other body part. Hence it does not display any color of bruise on external examination. However the swelling is very obvious as scrotum has more amount of loose connective tissue.

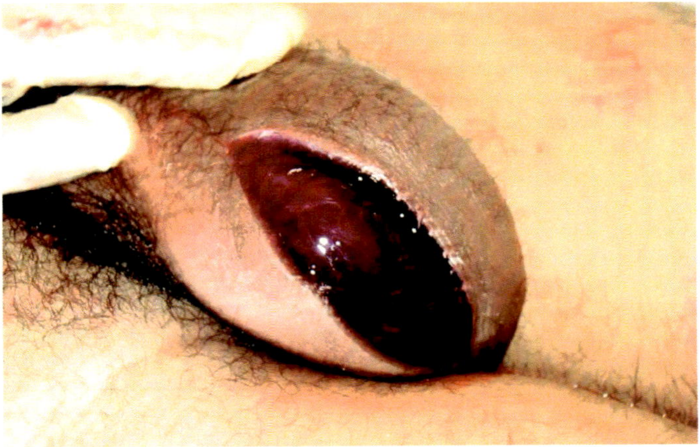

FIGURE 5.5: On dissection of scrotum in Figure 5.4 it revealed the extravasation of blood in scrotal loose connective tissue.

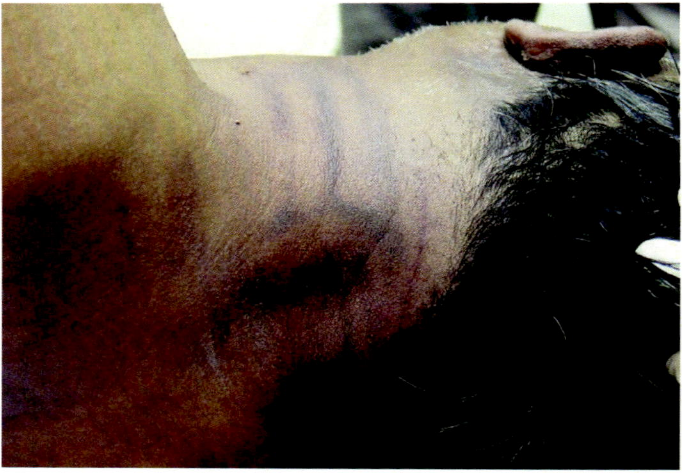

FIGURE 5.6: The bruise may not be visible on the site of impact. The extravasated blood may follow the gravitational force and get collected on the dependent part of body. As in this case the victim of head injury had a bruise in the scalp. However the colors of bruise were displayed on the nape of neck as he was hospitalized and bed ridden for about a week after sustaining the head injury.

The term 'Contusion' is used when the injuries are confined to the internal organs, e.g. brain, liver, spleen, lungs, heart, stomach, intestine, mesentery, urinary bladder, kidney, etc. In this case the contusion does not take the routine color changes with advancing age of that injury.

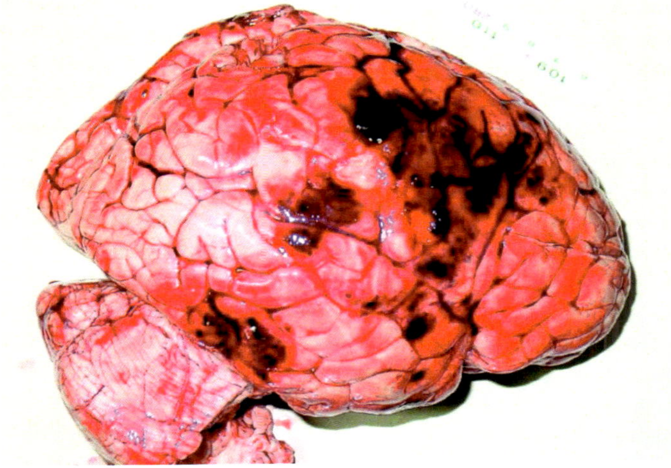

FIGURE 5.7: Contusions to brain. They are usually red to dark red for many days. They can be present at the site of impact (coup injury) or opposite to the site of impact (counter-coup injury) to brain.

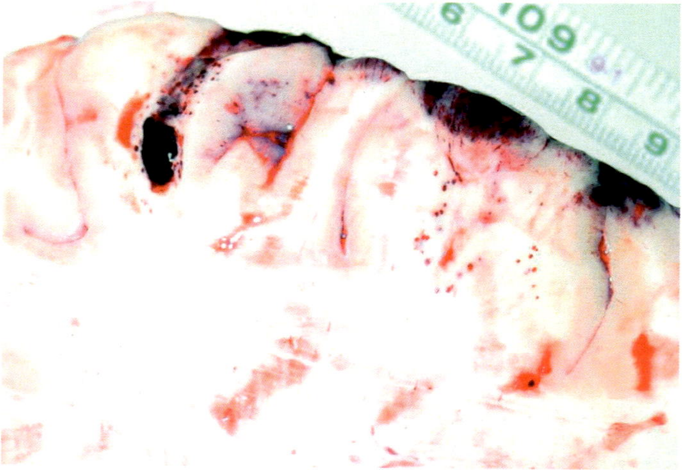

FIGURE 5.8: The cut section of the contusion of brain shows the extravasation of blood in grey matter.

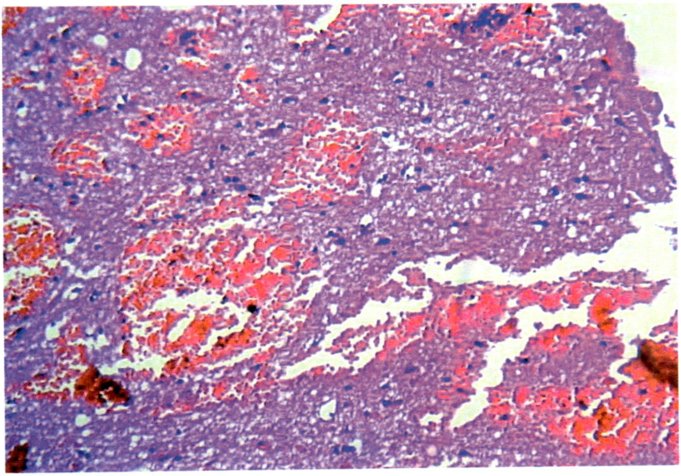

FIGURE 5.9: Whenever the age of a contusion or bruise is disputed, it is always bette- to go for histological study. This figure shows a recent contusion to brain. Note there are no recognizable blood pigments (X100 H and E stain).

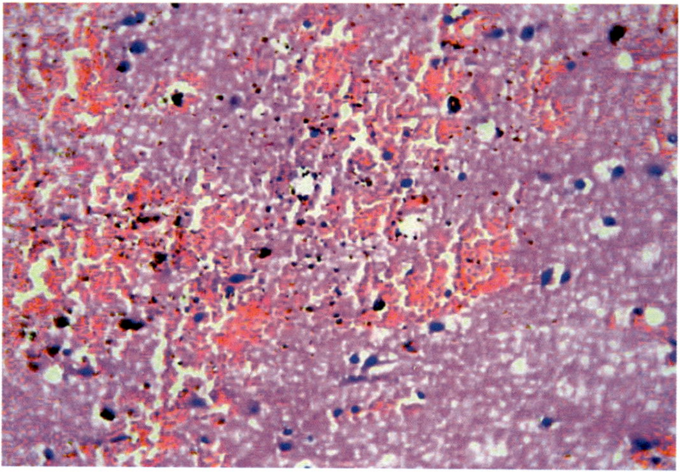

FIGURE 5.10: Old contusion of brain. Note the recognizable hemosiderin pigments (X400 H and E stain). However they must be confirmed by Perls' Prussian blue staining.

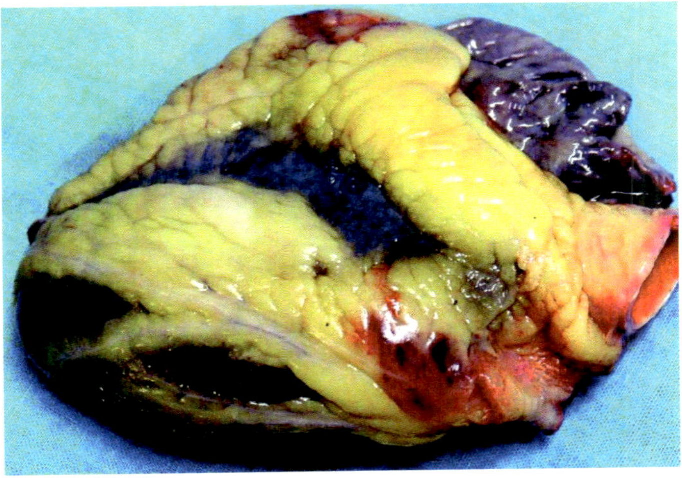

FIGURE 5.11: A recent contusion to heart. For appreciation of the contusions to organs having color either red or shades of red must be cleaned in running water.

When mechanical injury is caused to the superficial layer of the skin then it is called as abrasion. These injuries are strictly confined to the skin and they are caused by either crushing or tangential force.

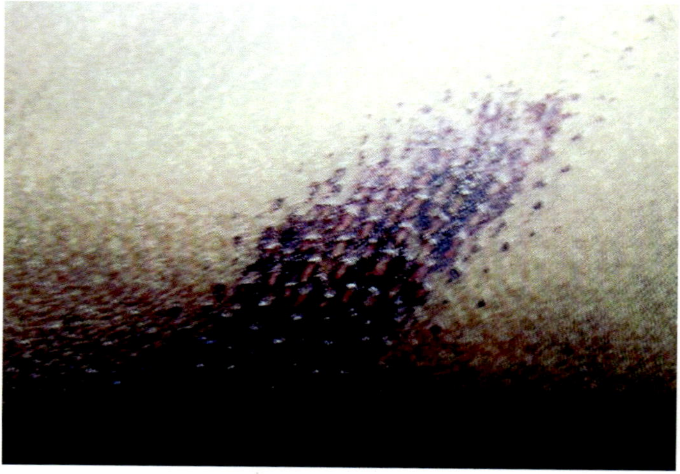

FIGURE 5.12: An abrasion caused by tangential force is called as graze. Note there is no 'true bleeding' from the injury as the superficial layer does not contain any blood vessels.

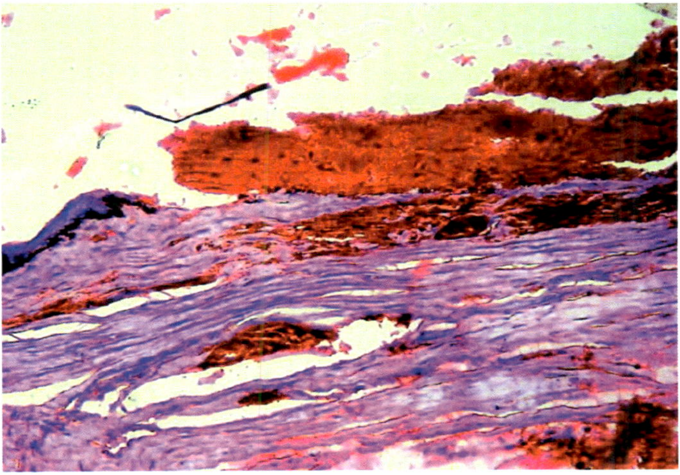

FIGURE 5.13: Many times the deeper layer of the skin is also involved as in this recent abrasion where the upper layer of skin is lost and blood cells are visible on external surface (X100 H and E stain).

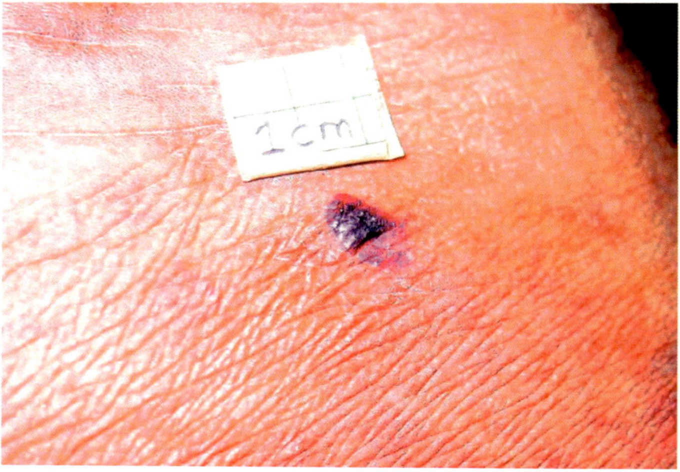

FIGURE 5.14: Sometimes the abrasion may be displayed as a vesicle. As in this case the abrasion is caused by striking of a returned kick pedal of the bike on the region of left medial malleolus. Note the blood tinged fluid in the vesicle.

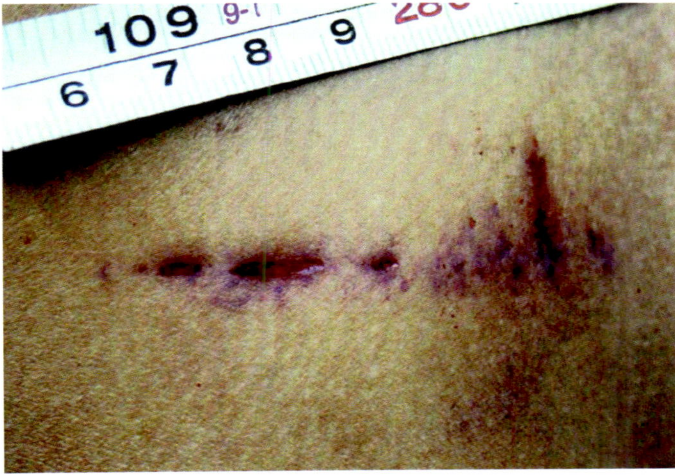

FIGURE 5.15: Abrasions caused by compression by compressing nails. Note the bruising in surrounding area. Pattern of abrasion depends on the fact that whether they are along or perpendicular to skin creases.

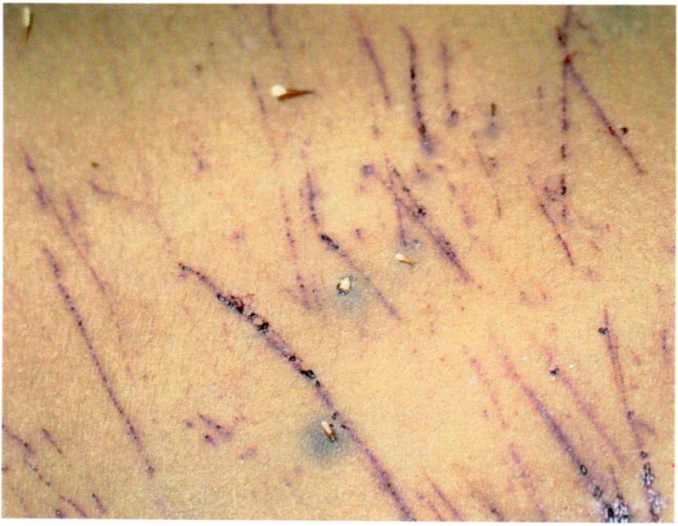

FIGURE 5.16: Scratch abrasions caused by thorns. Note the thorns *in situ* and bruise is present where the thorns are penetrated up to deeper layers of skin.

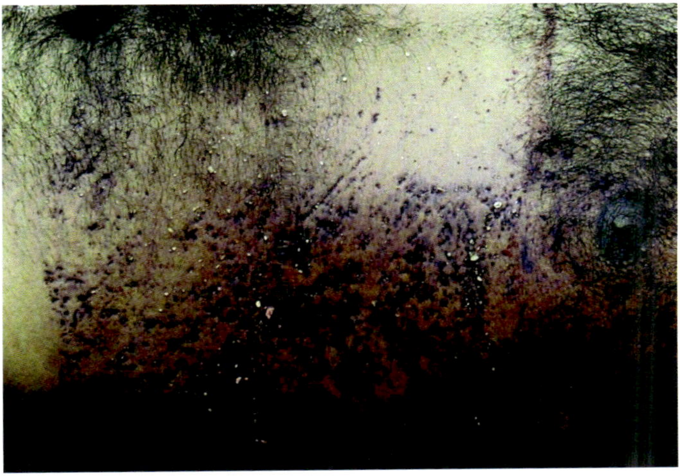

FIGURE 5.17: Impact abrasions caused by sand particles. Note the sand particles *in situ*.

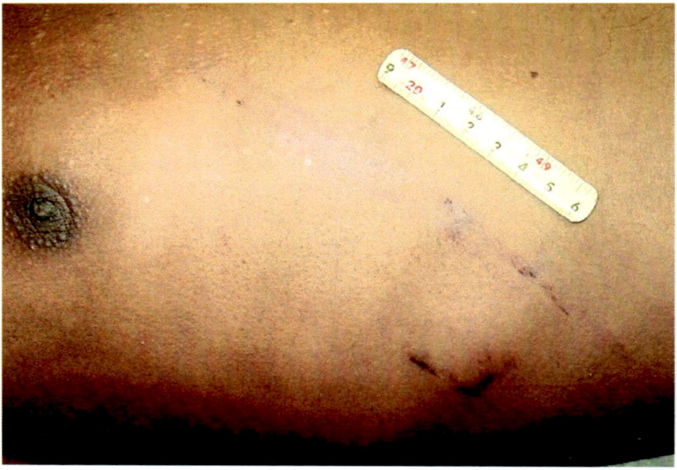

FIGURE 5.18: When the abrasion depicts the imprint of the causative agent then it is called as imprint abrasion. In this case the abrasion is caused by the impact of the edge of a wooden plank. Also note the imprint bruise in the same area of abrasion. Abrasion and contusion may be seen in combination many times.

When tissues get torn due to compression and crushing by the blunt force the resultant injury is laceration or lacerated wound or crush injury. Usually the tissues get crushed between the causative object and the underlying bone. Hence lacerations are commonly situated over the body parts where bones are superficial.

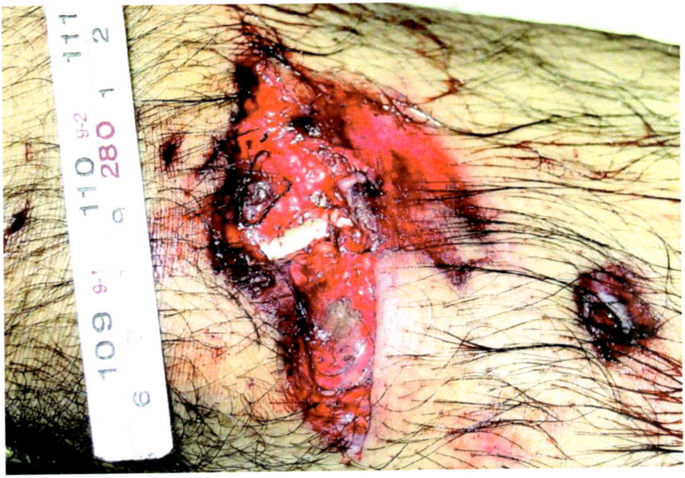

FIGURE 5.19: Lacerations have irregular, contused or abraded margins. Foreign bodies found in these injuries are very important clues to solve crimes. In this laceration over upper part of left sheen paint flak of the vehicle was found, which was used for identification of the vehicle. An intact vessel can also be noted in the small laceration.

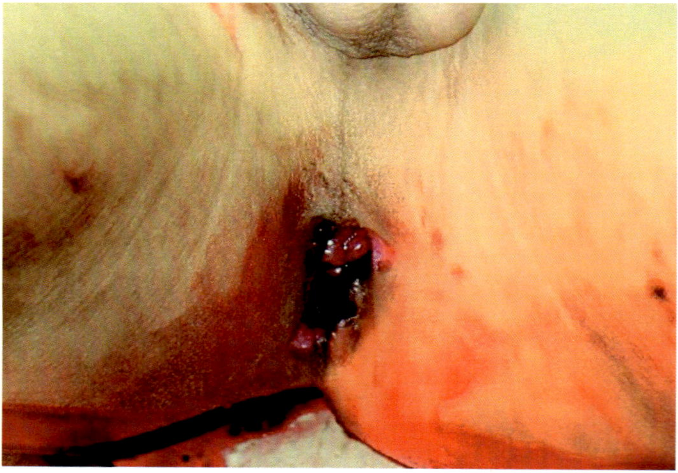

FIGURE 5.20: Lacerations can also be caused by stretching the tissue in two or more opposite directions. In such cases lacerations may be present over any site of the body. This laceration of anus is caused by stretching of both lower limbs in opposite direction. This type of laceration does not show any abrasion or contusion in their edges.

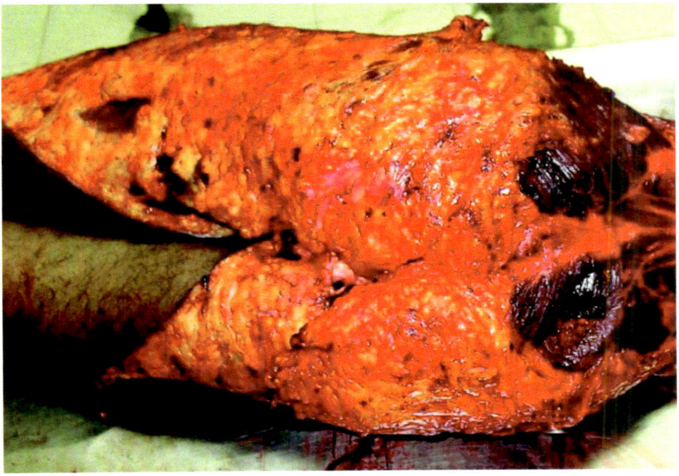

FIGURE 5.21: Sometimes the skin and underlying tissue may get lacerated and collected at one end due to tangential blunt force, such laceration is denoted as avulsion. The avulsion injury in the present figure is caused by the wheel of vehicle in a run over injury.

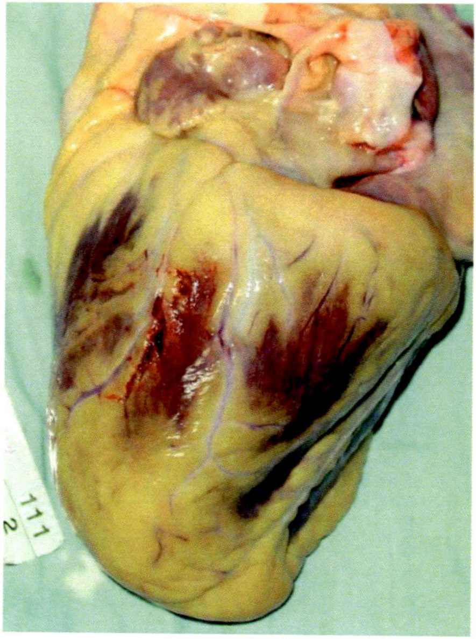

FIGURE 5.22: Lacerations of the internal organs can be found as blunt force injuries when they are present subjacent to site of impact. When present at areas other than the site of impact they are denoted as ruptures. In this case the heart was lacerated by subjacent bodies of thoracic vertebrae.

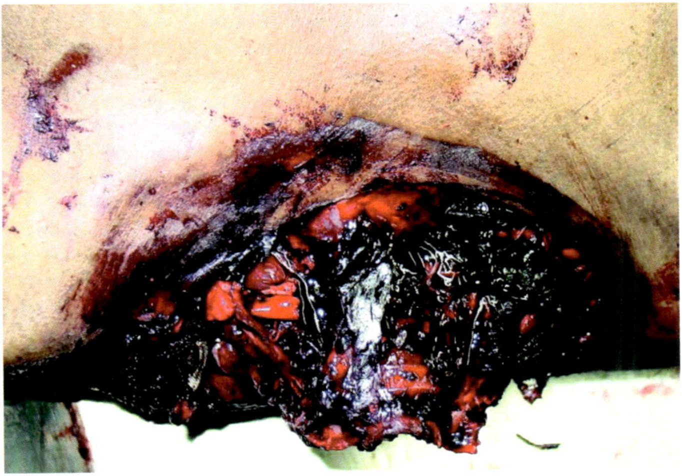

FIGURE 5.23: The extremely severe lacerations are crush injuries. Here the underlying structures are almost completely destroyed. The crushing usually occurs between two blunt objects with direction of force towards each other. This is a photograph of crush decapitation injury caused by crushing between rail track and train wheel. Note the abraded surrounding area of the wound caused by the rim of train wheel. Grease stains are commonly found around such injuries.

Fracture is mechanical injury which is caused to the bones or cartilages. Blunt force is responsible for almost all fractures. However they can be caused by cutting or penetrating forces.

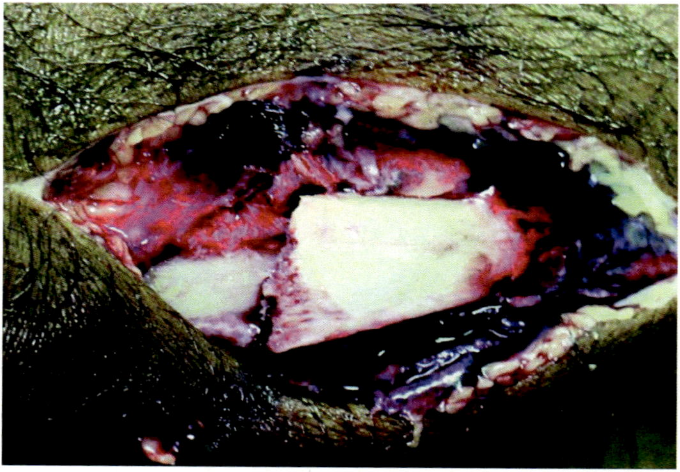

FIGURE 5.24: A recent fracture of a long bone showing disruption and extravasation of blood in the surrounding tissue.

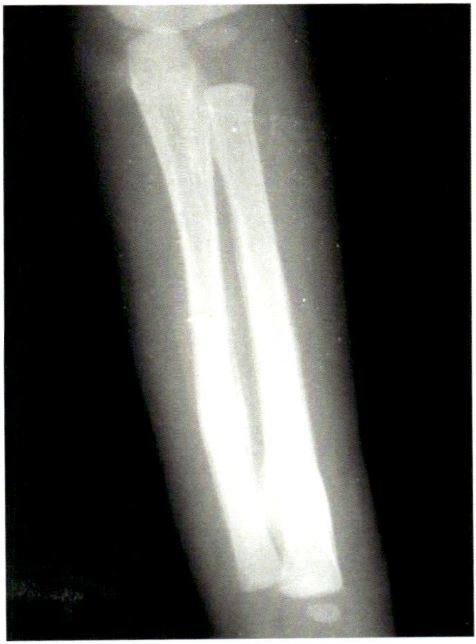

FIGURE 5.25: Whole body radiography is recommended in cases of death due to battered baby syndrome or battered wife syndrome or cases with history of torture or repeated physical abuse to identify fractures and to determine their age. However the age of the injury must be decided on the basis of gross, X-ray, histological examination and the history supplied as none of them signal a foolproof method to determine age. As in this X- ray photograph there is radiologically detectable hard callus at fracture of the radius and periosteal reaction around fractured ulna.

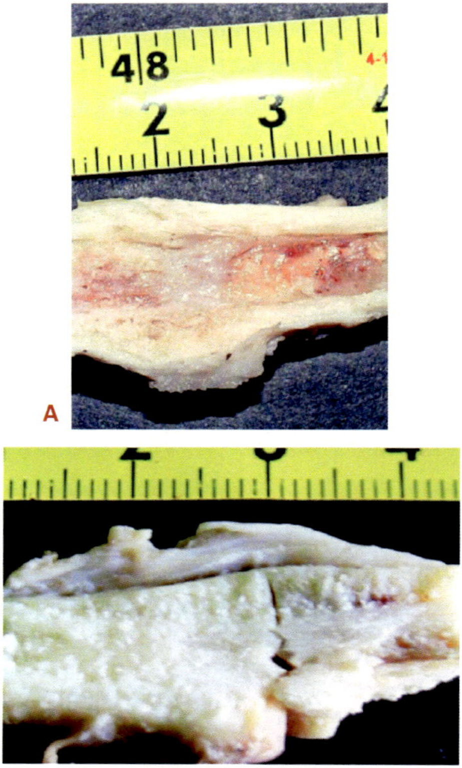

FIGURES 5.26A AND B: However gross examination of both fractured site revealed hard callus. These are longitudinal sections of the fractured site. (Photographed after fixation of tissue in 10% formalin for 3 days).

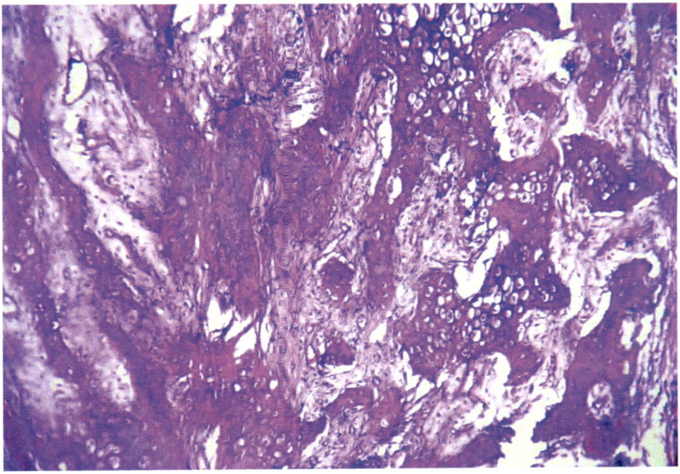

FIGURE 5.27: Histological examination of both fracture sites revealed callus formation with fibrosis, granulation tissue, cartilage and new bone formation indicating that both the fractures are of about same age (X100 H and E stain).

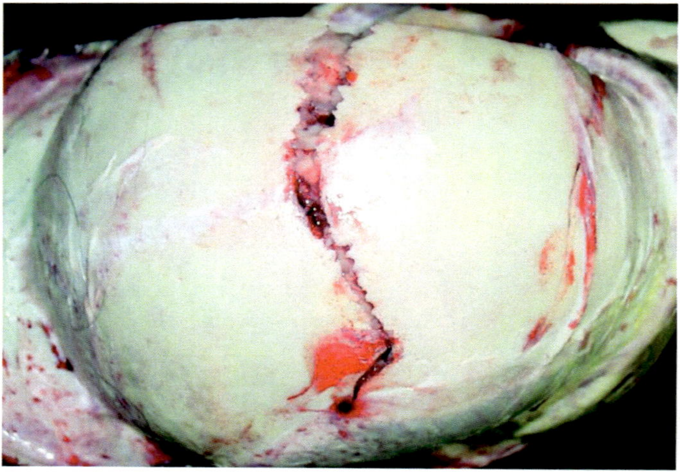

FIGURE 5.28: There are different types of fractures of skull, e.g. this photograph shows a fractured suture. Healing process of the skull and cartilage fractures are entirely different than the healing of fractured long bone.

INJURIES CAUSED BY CUTTING FORCE (FIGS 5.29 TO 5.35)

Cutting edge of a weapon either causes an incised wound or chop wound. In incised wound the length of the injury is always greater than its depth. Chop wounds are usually caused by sharp edged heavy weapon.

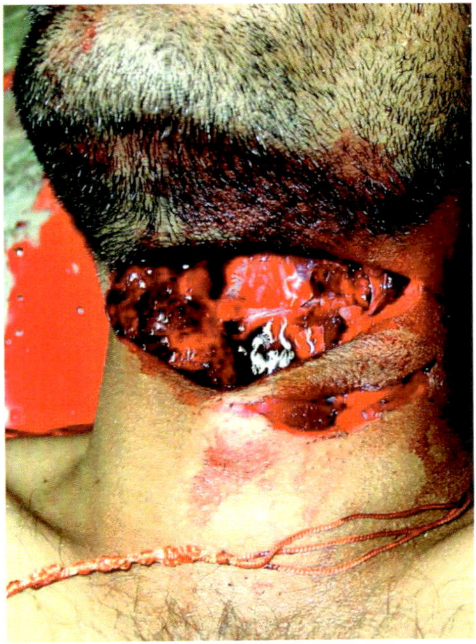

FIGURE 5.29: A homicidal cut throat injury caused by a sharp cutting knife. Note the cut on the anterior surface of body of the cervical vertebrae. Tailing of the incised wound is that end of the wound from where the weapon is drawn-out. The depth becomes shallower till it ends in a linear abrasion. However when the incised wounds are present on the more rounded part of the body e.g. neck, fingers, arms, etc. it is very difficult to determine which one is the tailing end as they are apparently shallow on both ends.

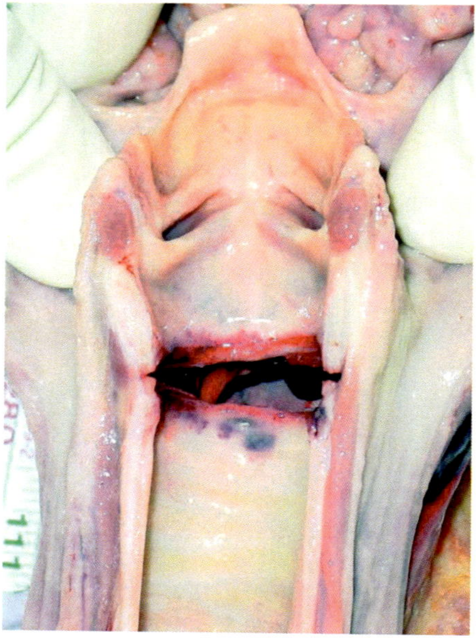

FIGURE 5.30: Note completely cut larynx at the level of cricoid cartilage caused by a knife. Note that the inner lining of the larynx is retracted from cut injury.

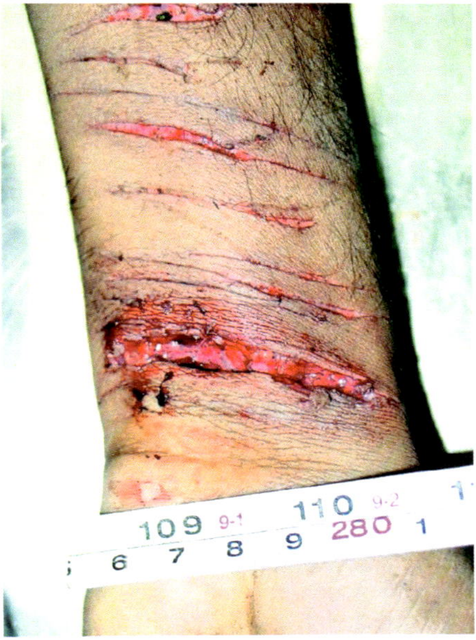

FIGURE 5.31: Suicidal cr self inflicted incised wounds are usually seen on approachable parts of the body and opposite to the handedness of the person. They are superficial, parallel and unidirectional, i.e. tailing in one direction. These are self-inflicted incised wounds over anterior lower third of left forearm and wrist in a right handed person.

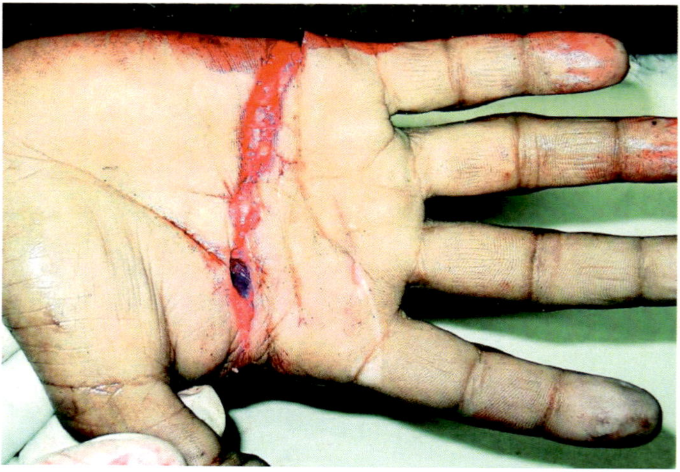

FIGURE 5.32: When a victim tries to protect himself by holding the cutting blade of weapon or try to protect his vital parts of body by covering those parts with hands, forearms and/or arms, the injuries sustained by him over outer surface of those parts are called as defense wounds.

The edges of the chop wound are frequently contused and abraded. The underlying bone is usually cut fractured.

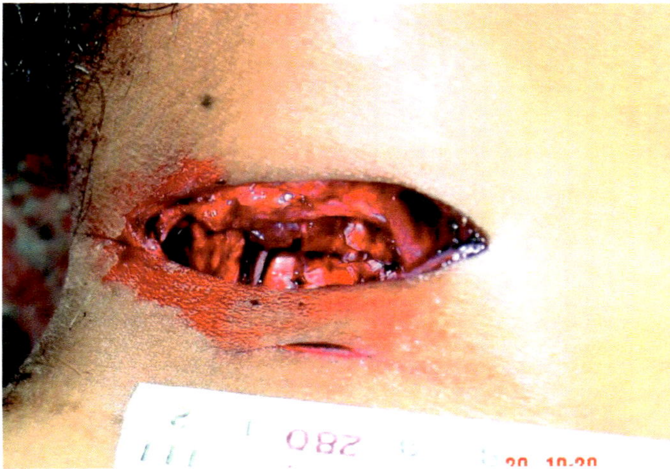

FIGURE 5.33: A chop wound caused by axe (Parashu). Note the underlying cut fracture of bone.

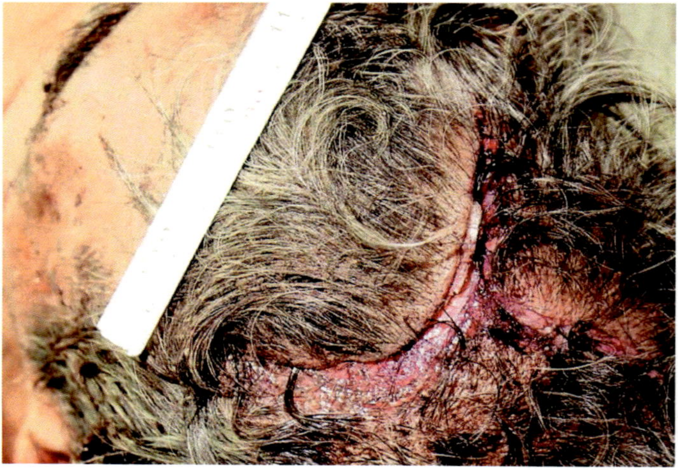

FIGURE 5.34: A chop wound caused by tangential blow of the blade of a sword over head.

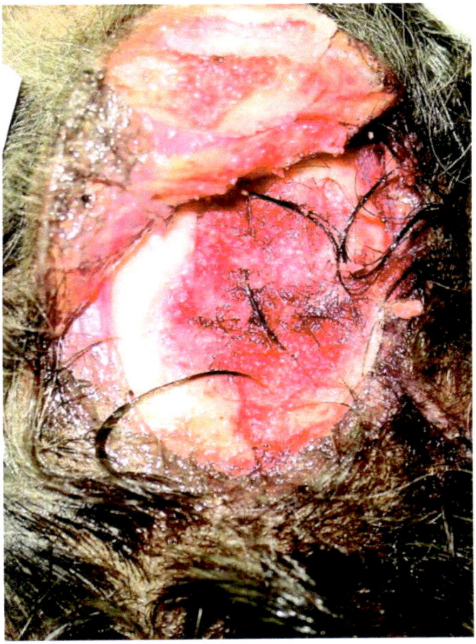

FIGURE 5.35: Opening the wound in Figure 5.34 revealed the cutting of the outer table of the skull.

INJURIES CAUSED BY THRUSTING FORCE (FIGS 5.36 TO 5.40)

In injuries caused by thrusting force, if the depth of the injury is greater than the length of the injury, it is called a penetrating or stab wound. They are fatal if they penetrate the body cavity and cause damage to the internal viscera or artery. When the wound has entry and exit wound then it is called as perforating injury.

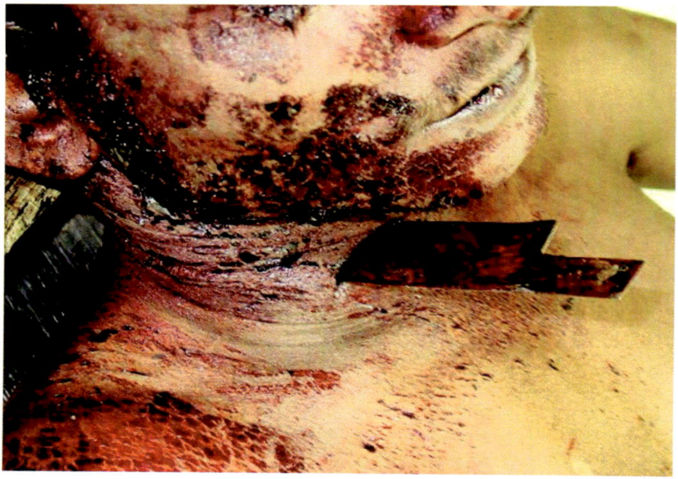

FIGURE 5.36: A stab wound caused by thrusting of a sharp edged blade. Externally they are pear or elliptical in shape. Here the weapon is *in situ*.

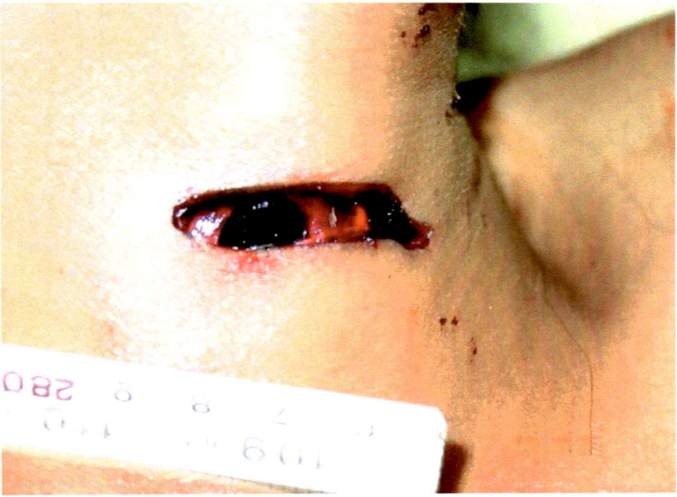

FIGURE 5.37: Note the ends or angles of the stab after removal of the weapon.

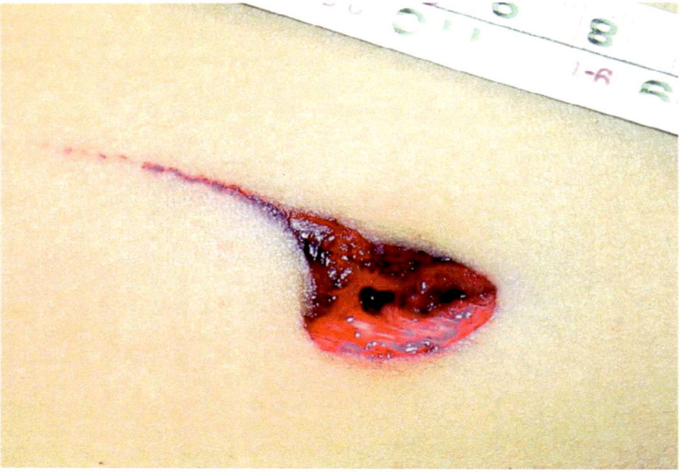

FIGURE 5.38: When the thrusted blade of the weapon is taken out with decreasing angulation the stab injury gets an additional feature at the end 'tailing'.

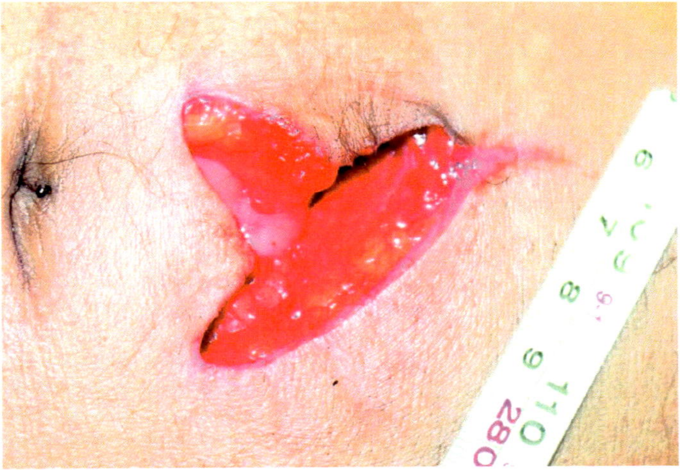

FIGURE 5.39: When the weapon is rotated or rocked in the body after thrusting it gives rise to three or four ends or angles depending on at which axis the blade was rotated.

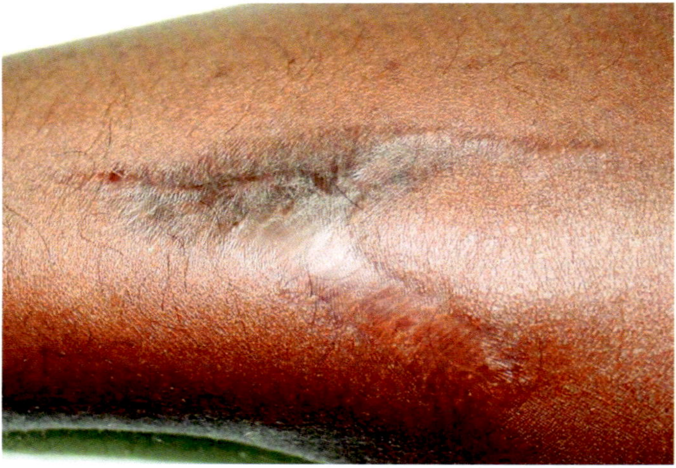

FIGURE 5.40: Dating or age of wound can be inferred from presence of bleeding, clot, infection, and granulation tissue and scaring. This is an old scar of injury caused by a spear.

INJURIES CAUSED BY FIREARMS (FIGS 5.41 TO 5.53)

Firearm injuries are caused due to missiles fired from firearms. Their characteristics depends on the type of firearm i.e. whether it is a smooth-bore or rifled weapon, distance between the body surface and muzzle end of barrel, the type of cartridge, the media through which the missile travels before hitting the body and the body part which is struck by the missile.

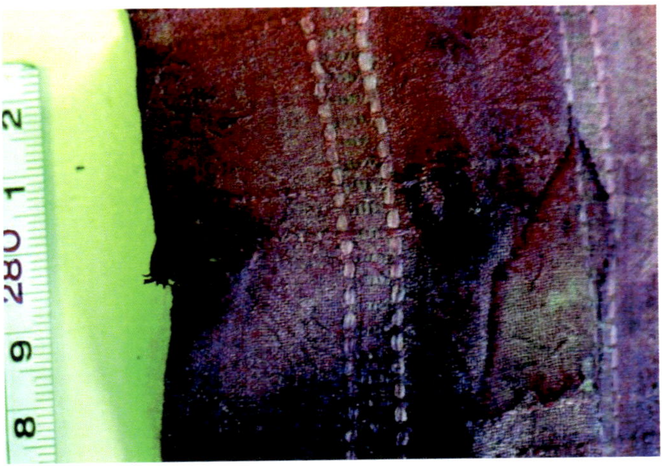

FIGURE 5.41: The clothes damaged in a close range accidental fire of a revolver. Note the blackening and burning of the fabric around the rent. The border was folded on the area of rent at the time of firing.

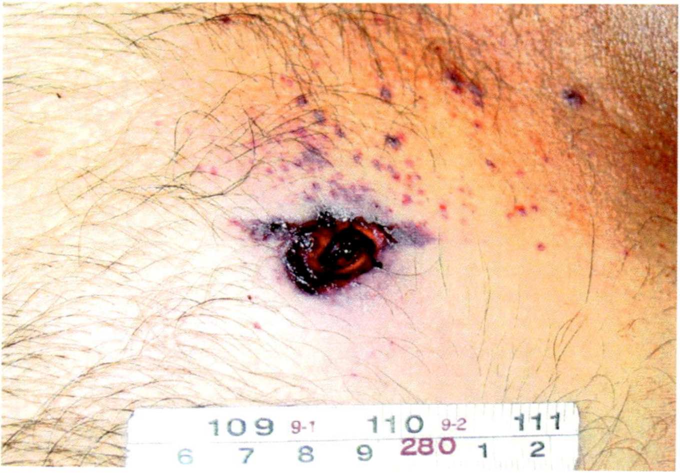

FIGURE 5.42: The close range firearm entry wound in same case. Note the stippling on the adjacent area which was not covered and the abrasion caused by the forceful entry of cloth in the entry wound.

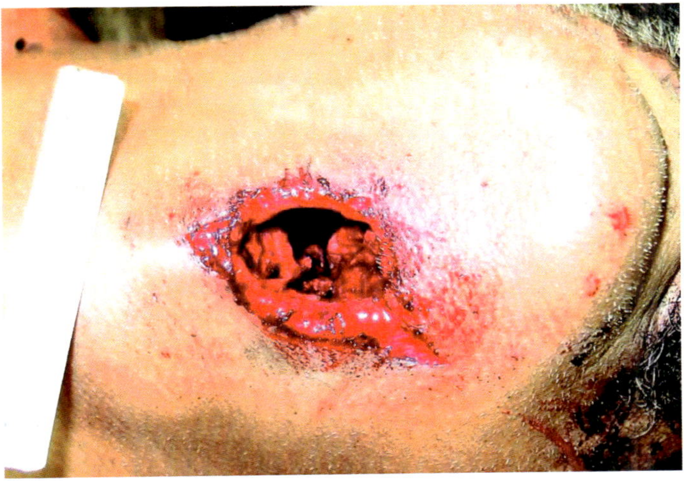

FIGURE 5.43: A contact entry wound made by a service pistol. Note the shape caused due to blast effect.

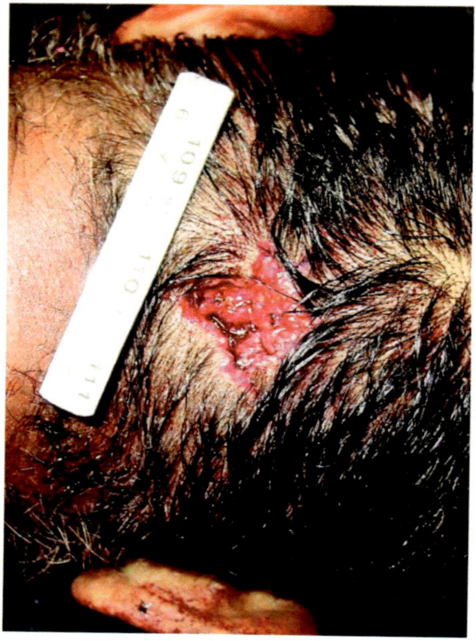

FIGURE 5.44: The exit wound in the same case.

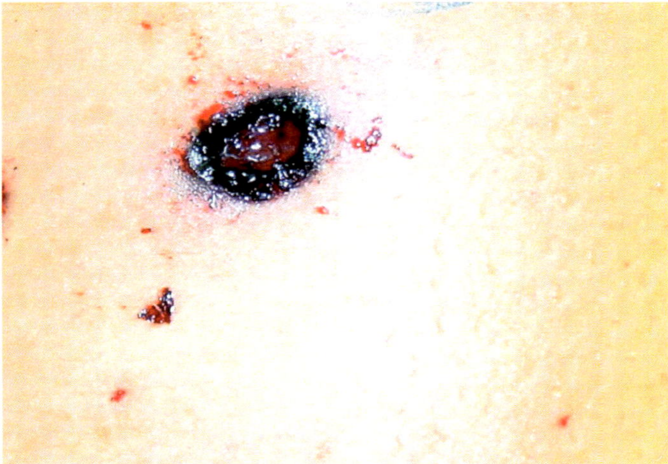

FIGURE 5.45: The distant range firearm entry wound from firing of a pistol. Note the abrasion collar.

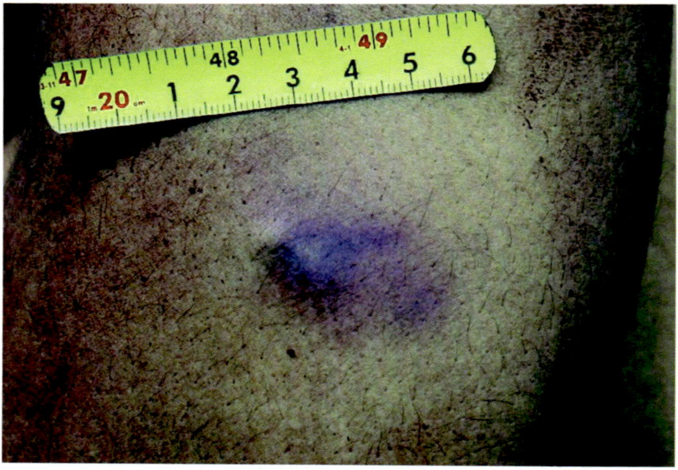

FIGURE 5.46: Sometimes the bullet can be palpated if it is lodged below skin.

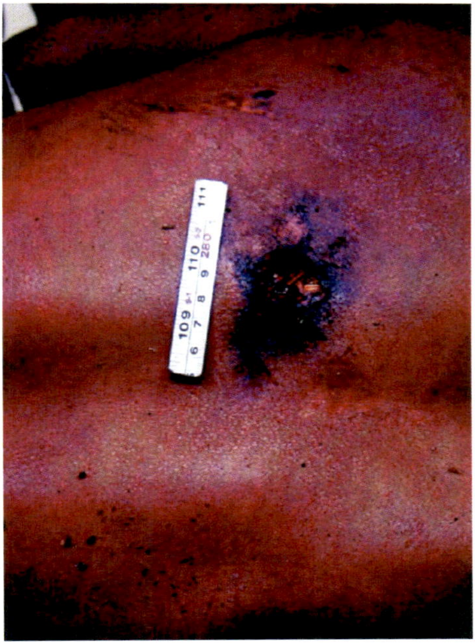

FIGURE 5.47: A close range entry wound by a shotgun firing. Note the soiling and stippling on the surrounding skin.

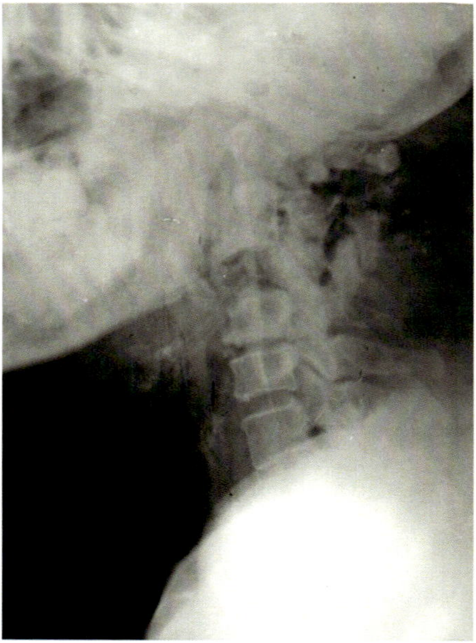

FIGURE 5.48: Radiography is very much necessary in cases of firearm injury to define the damage and locate the missile. This is X-ray of neck and head (lateral view) in the case depicted in Figures 5.43 and 5.44 where the direction of path of bullet and damage caused can be easily demonstrated.

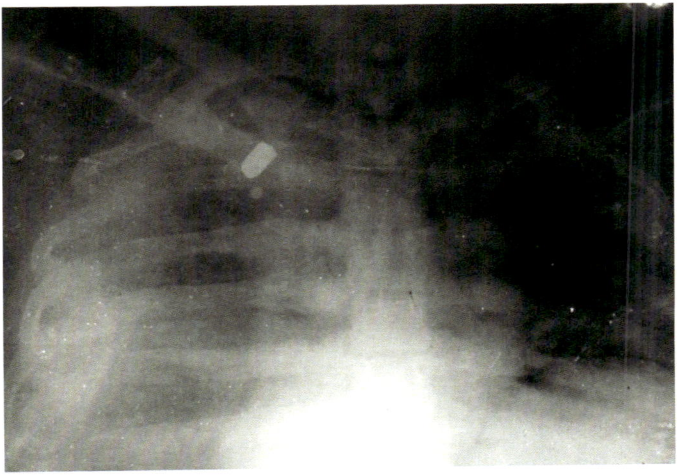

FIGURE 5.49: Radiography can reveal the situation of the missile.

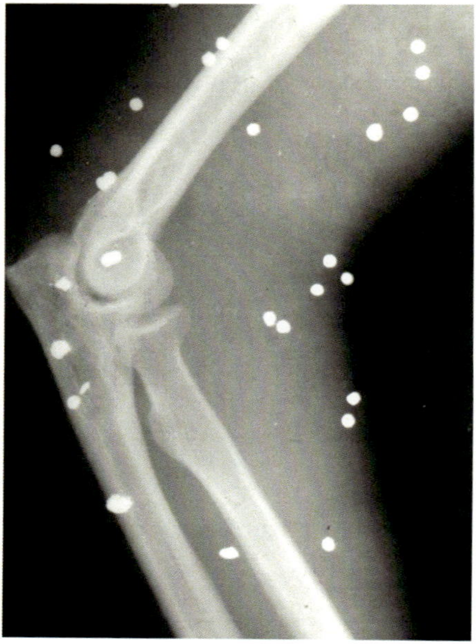

FIGURE 5.50: Radiography can also reveal the span of pellets sprayed.

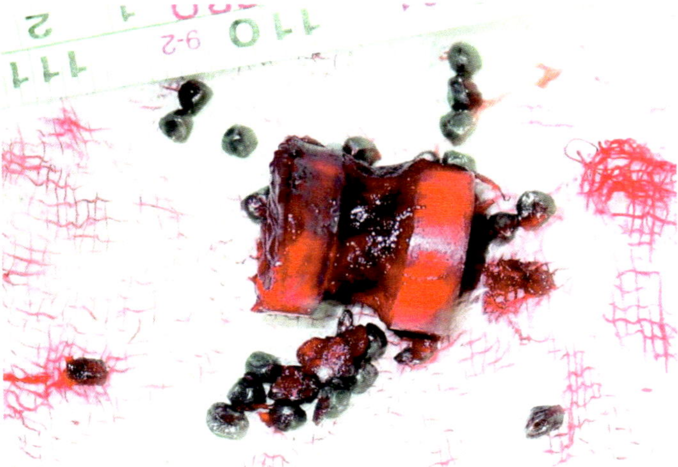

FIGURE 5.51: The pellets and wad removed from a close range firearm injury. They must be removed carefully; air dried without washing and packed in a gauge piece and cardboard box before sending to ballistic expert.

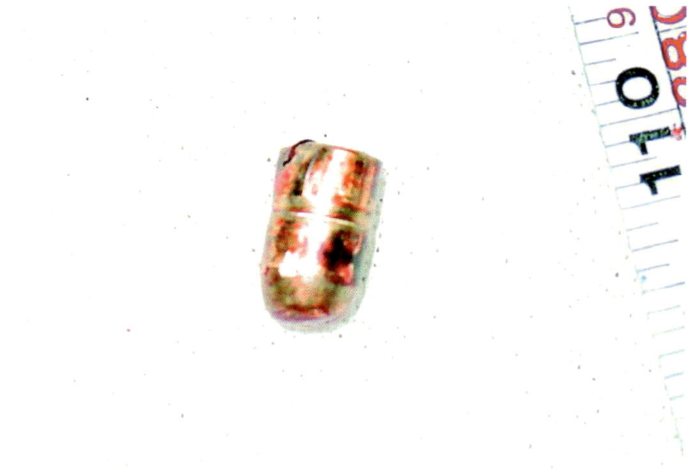

FIGURE 5.52: The bullet must not be removed or handled by forceps. After removal it must not be kept or dropped on hard surface like kidney tray. It must not be washed or cleaned or rubbed by cloth or paper, as all these procedures may distort the signature of firearm on the bullet. It is best to remove it with fingertips, kept it on a gauge piece, air dried and packed in gauge piece followed by cardboard box, before sending it to the ballistic expert.

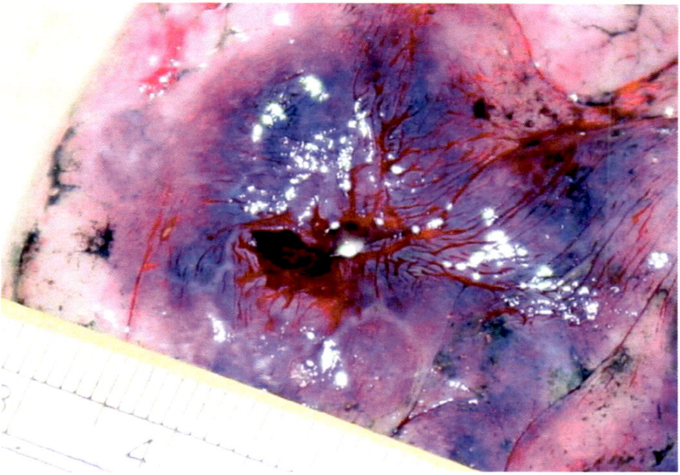

FIGURE 5.53: It must always be remembered that a bullet fired from rifled weapon not only causes a rent in the organ when it travels through that organ but also damages a huge circumferential area due to acquired centrifugal force from gyratory motion of the bullet and negative pressure created at the rear end of the bullet. Here although the rent in the lung is small but the huge surrounding damaged area can be seen.

INJURIES CAUSED BY BOMB BLAST (FIGS 5.54 AND 5.55)

Injuries caused by bomb blast depend on the type of explosive material, its range and distance of the victim from the blast site.

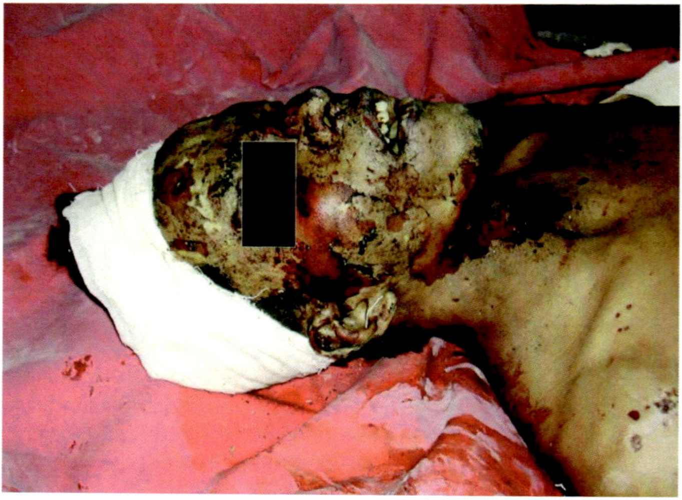

FIGURE 5.54: The photograph reveals penetrating injuries with burns indicating that the victim was within the range of flames of the blast as missiles produced by a blast travels further than flames.

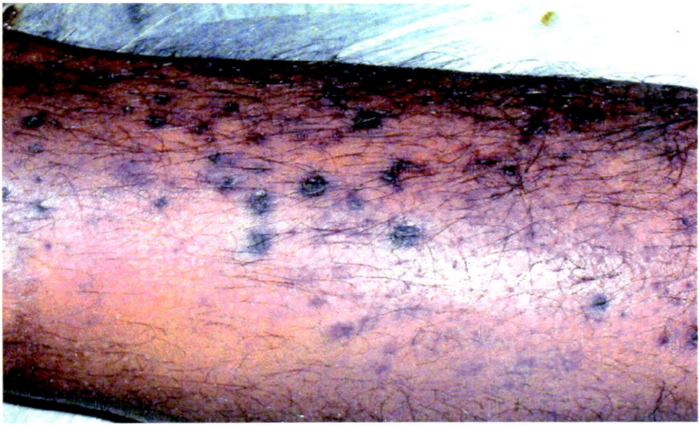

FIGURE 5.55: As this victim was beyond the reach of flames of bomb blast, there were only penetrating injuries, that too on the body part which was not covered by cloths and facing the blast site. (Figures 5.54 and 5 55 *Courtesy*: Dr Sanjay Deoba Wathore, Chief Medical Officer, Mumbai Central Prison, Arthur Road Jail, Mumbai).

TRAUMATIC INTRACRANIAL HEMORRHAGES (FIGS 5.56 TO 5.58)

There are three brain coverings/meninges.

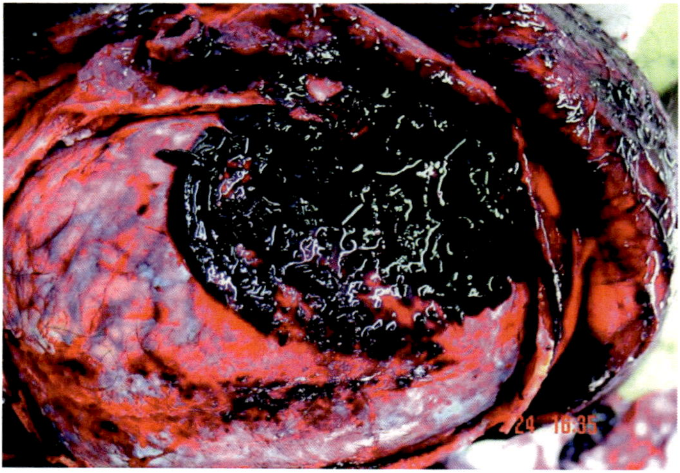

FIGURE 5.56: Dura mater, the outermost covering of brain which is firmly attached to the skull from inside. Middle meningeal artery and their tributaries lies between dura and skull. As they lie in the grooves made by them on the inner surface of skull they are well protected from diseases and trauma. However whenever they are traumatized the blood get collected between dura and skull known as extradural hematoma. When this hematoma is caused due to rupture of vein, it is small and many times asymptomatic if the victim is alive. This hematoma may be caused due to trauma to dural sinuses.

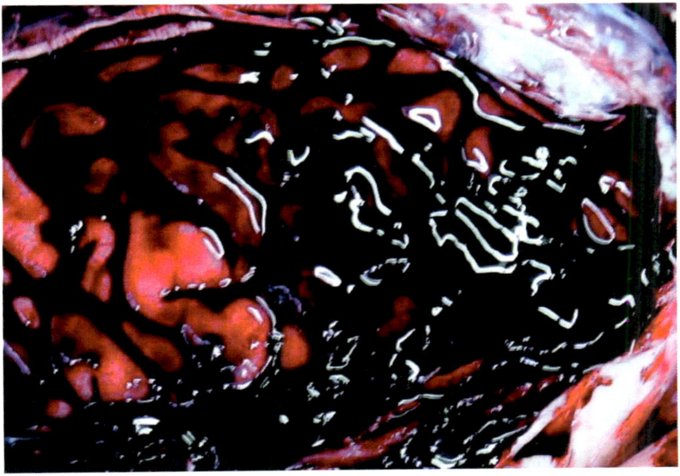

FIGURE 5.57: The arachnoid matter is the second and middle covering of the brain. The bleeding due to trauma above and below this covering is commonly caused due to laceration of superior cerebral veins. When the bleeding occurs above this covering then it is called as subdural hemorrhage or hematoma. When the bleeding occurs below this covering in the cerebrospinal fluid then it is known as subarachnoid hemorrhage. Subarachnoid hemorrhages can also be caused due to trauma to spine and spinal cord and trauma to vertebral artery above the level of its entrance in this space. Both the hemorrhages are possible by contusion or laceration of brain. Chronic subdural hematoma is encapsulated and adherent to dura mater due to formation of neomembrane.

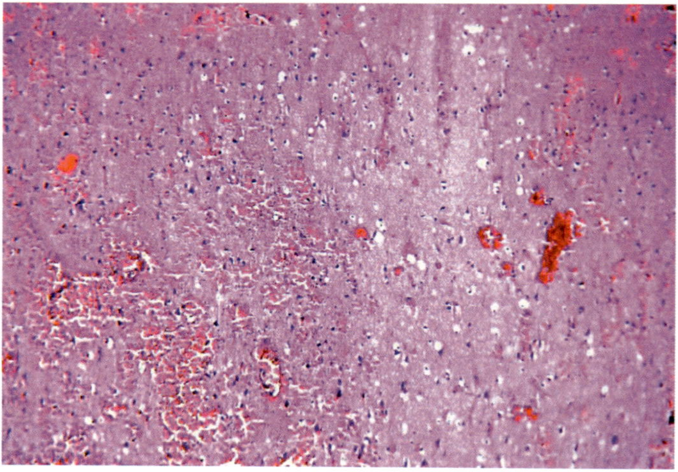

FIGURE 5.58: Traumatic intracerebral hemorrhages are very common. They occur in gray matter and extend in white matter. This microphotograph shows traumatic intracerebral hemorrhages (X100 H and E stain).

6 Injuries by the Fire and Electricity

BURNS (FIGS 6.1 TO 6.22)

Burns and scalds are the thermal injuries caused by dry and moist heat respectively. The severity of the thermal injuries depends on the intensity of heat applied, time period of its application and the body parts involved. Burns can be seen as mere redness of skin or mucosa to complete consumption of the body part.

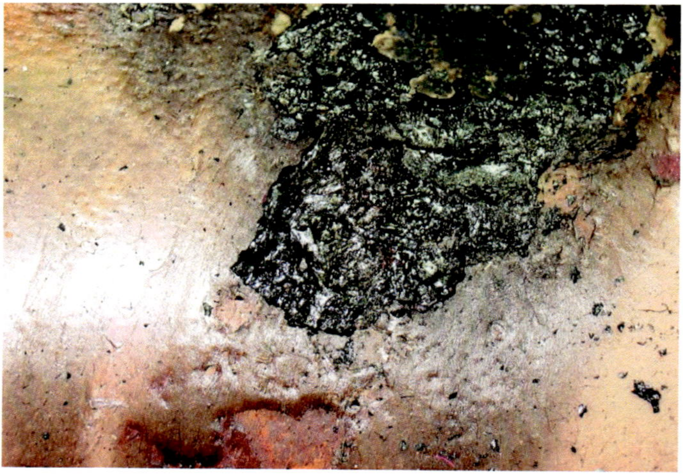

FIGURE 6.1: When the damages by fire are caused to the superficial layer of skin – epidermis then they look as red flared area. When the epidermis and upper layer of dermis is damaged by heat usually there is vesicle formation containing protein rich fluid. Burnt or un-burnt cloths adherent to body surface must be collected for detection of inflammable material or its residues on chemical analysis. Many hydrocarbons can be detected from completely burnt cloth if the inflammable material like petrol, diesel or kerosene oil is used in the process of burning.

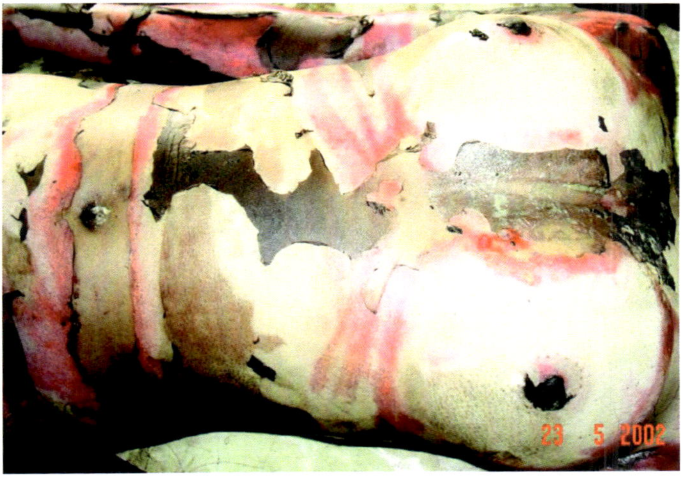

FIGURE 6.2: The red line of vital reaction is considered for labeling a burn as an antemortem burn. However it must be remembered that the red or dark red dermal burns indicate that only the upper layer dermis is involved and the elements of true skin are still present. On healing, this type of burns gives rise to scars without contractures. Pale color of the burnt area is caused due to involvement of deeper layer of dermis and complete loss of true elements of skin. On healing, this type of burn result into scaring with contracture.

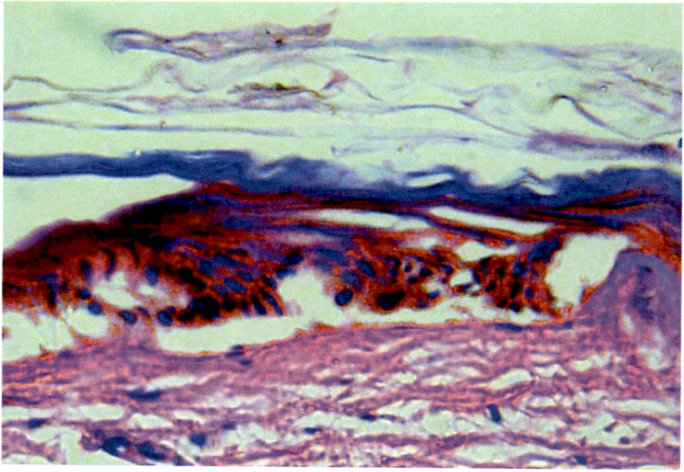

FIGURE 6.3: Microscopically the epidermal burns show the nuclear streaming and separation of epidermis due to heat (X100 H and E stain).

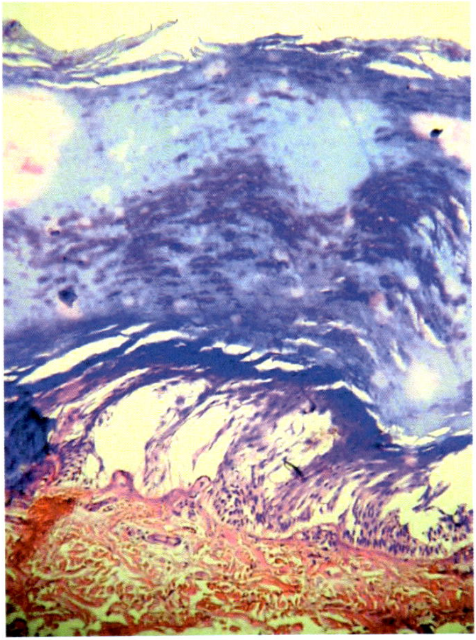

FIGURE 6.4: The microphotograph of burnt sole skin showing nuclear streaming, separation of epidermis due to heat and increased tissue eosinophilia (X100 H and E stain).

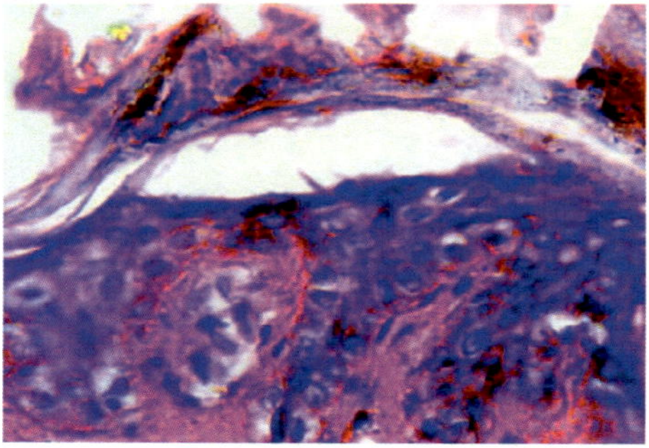

FIGURE 6.5A: Histology of a vesicle (X400 H and E stain).

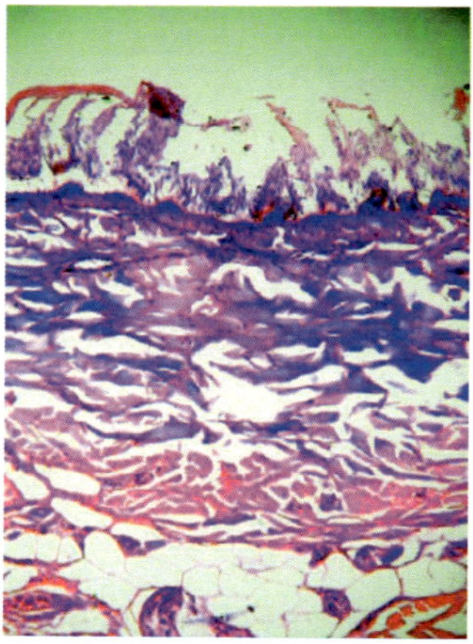

FIGURE 6.5B: Epidermis is damaged. The dermis is burnt and shows increased eosinophilia and separation of dermal layers (X400 H and E stain).

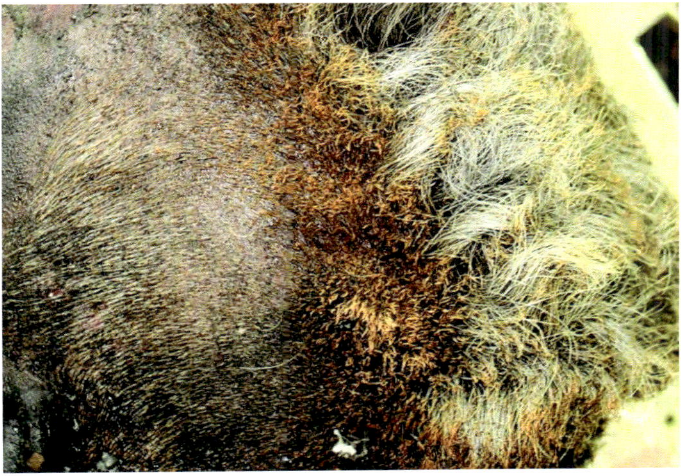

FIGURE 6.6: If the burns are caused by fire then it shows blackening, sooting and singeing of hair. These features are absent in burns caused by steam or hot water. Application of flame to gray hair turns the hair color to shades of yellow and red.

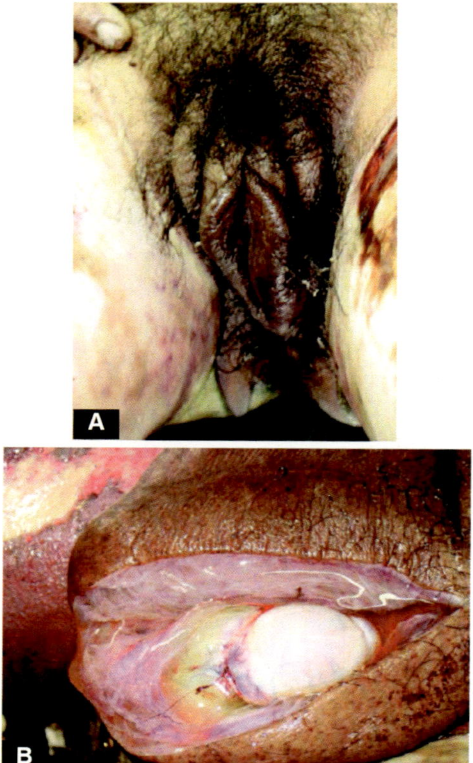

FIGURES 6.7A AND B: When the burn injuries are caused to the area of body where more amount of loose connective tissue is present in the subjacent area, such burnt area show large swelling of that region, e.g. external genitalia, eyelids, lips, etc.

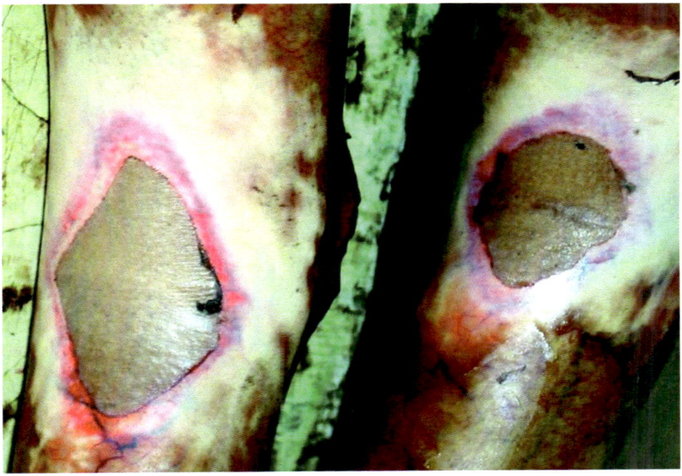

FIGURE 6.8: The body surfaces where the clothes are firmly adherent and the skin which is folded in the skin fold, e.g. axilla, popletial fossa, lower breast folds in female are spared from burn injury as the flame could not reach in those areas. Also denoted as 'shadow areas', in this case the knees of the victim was flexed while burning. Hence the poplitial areas were spared.

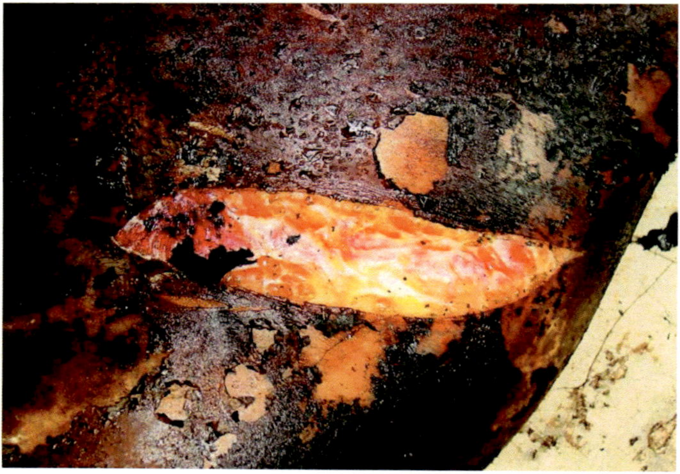

FIGURE 6.9: Intense heat application for longer period may cause coagulation of skin proteins which gives rise to splits or heat lacerations or heat ruptures. They do not bleed, nor show any vital reaction even though they are present when the victim is alive.

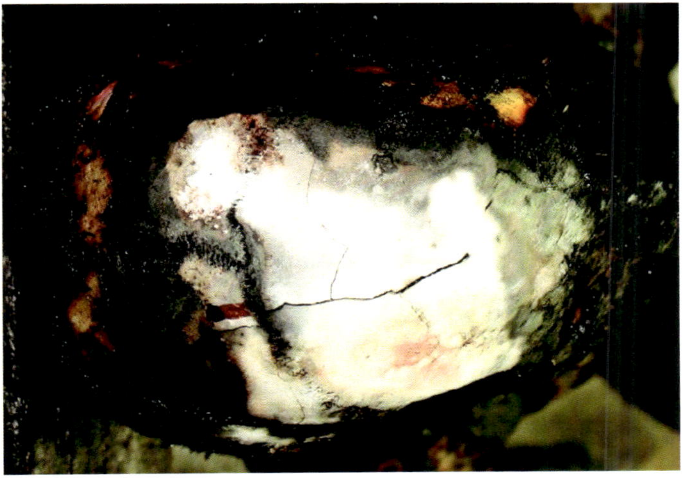

FIGURE 6.10: Application of intense heat for long time or incineration of head gives rise to complete charring of the scalp. When the skull vault is directly exposed to the flames, it desiccates and becomes chalky white to gray giving rise to multiple postmortem fractures.

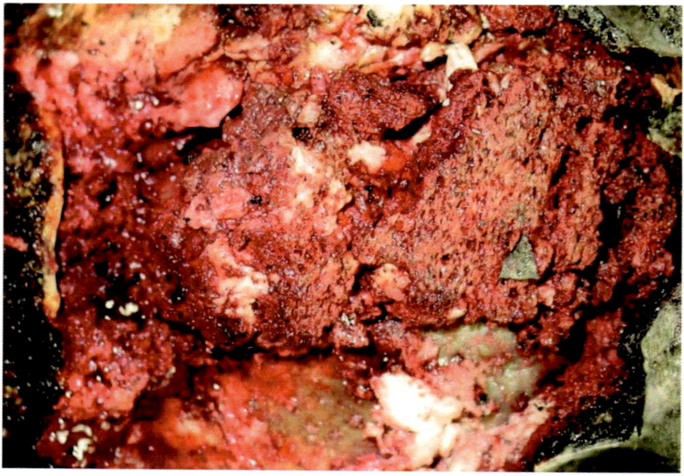

FIGURE 6.11: The blood may accumulate in the extradural space due to prolonged postmortem heating called as heat hematoma. It looks like sponge as it is formed by heat coagulation due to boiling of blood and they extend across the midline.

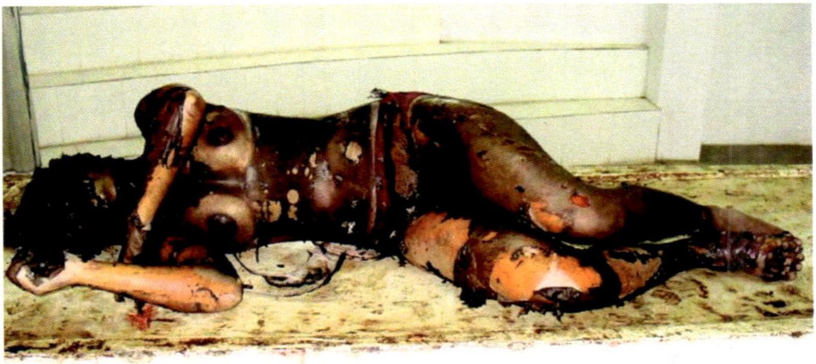

FIGURE 6.12: Pugilistic attitude or heat rigor occurs due to muscles stiffening and shortening as a result of prolonged postmortem exposure of body to heat. As the flexors are bulkier than extensors the joints become flexed.

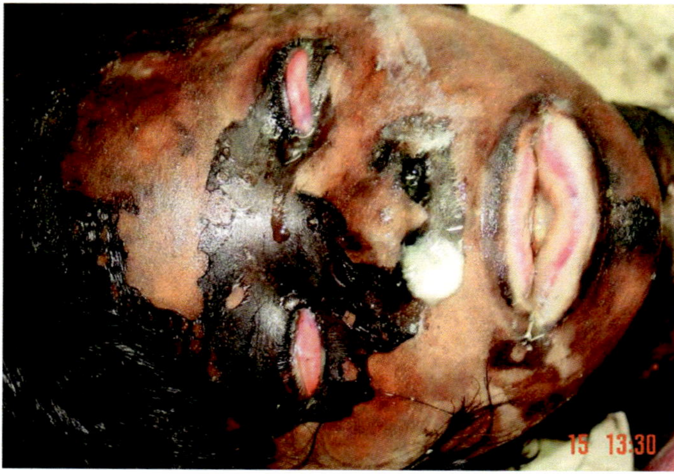

FIGURE 6.13: Burns are fatal when they are present over the face or around the mouth and nose or they are caused when the victim is burnt in a closed space. In these cases the victim may inhale hot fumes or air which causes burns to the respiratory tract. Note the edema of the conjunctiva, burns to lips and nostrils and froth from nostrils due to acute edema of lung.

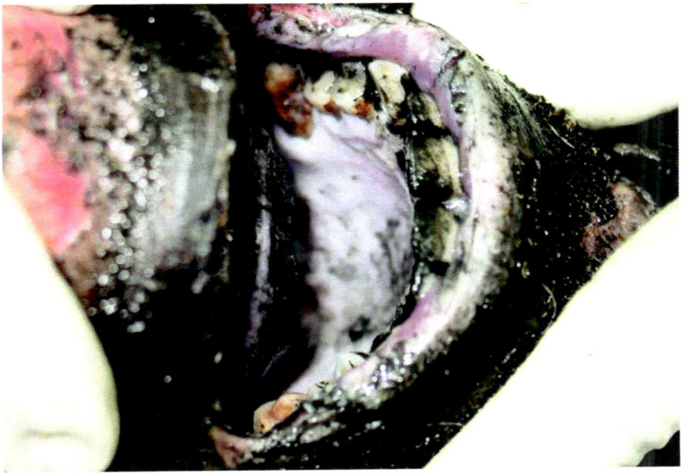

FIGURE 6.14: Deposition of soot over teeth, pallet and tongue are the common findings when the victim is breathing when burnt.

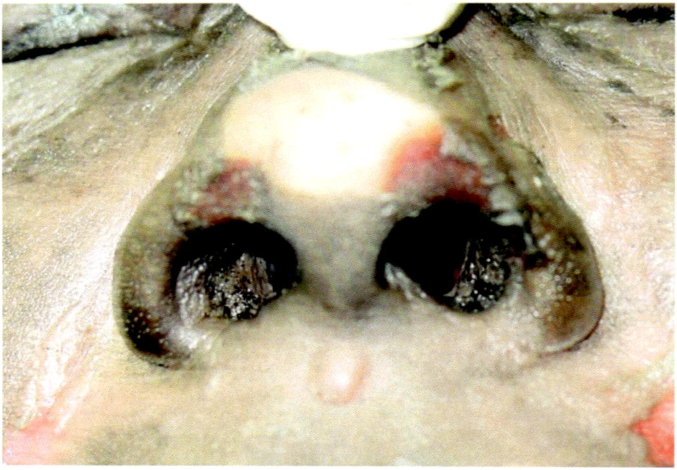

FIGURE 6.15: Singeing of hair in the nostrils, presence of soot mixed with mucus and scorching of nasal mucosa can be found if the victim was breathing hot fumes and flames through the nostrils.

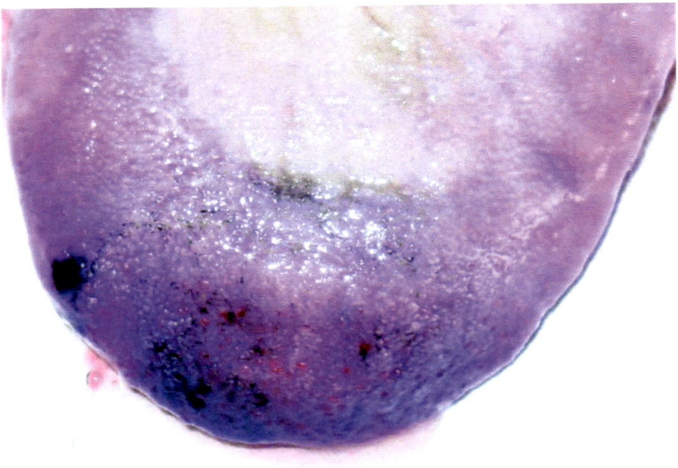

FIGURE 6.16: Protrusion and clinching of tongue between teeth is again a common finding in victims of burn and can be mistaken as caused due to strangulation. However, scorching of tongue and contusions caused by bite proves that the burns are antemortem.

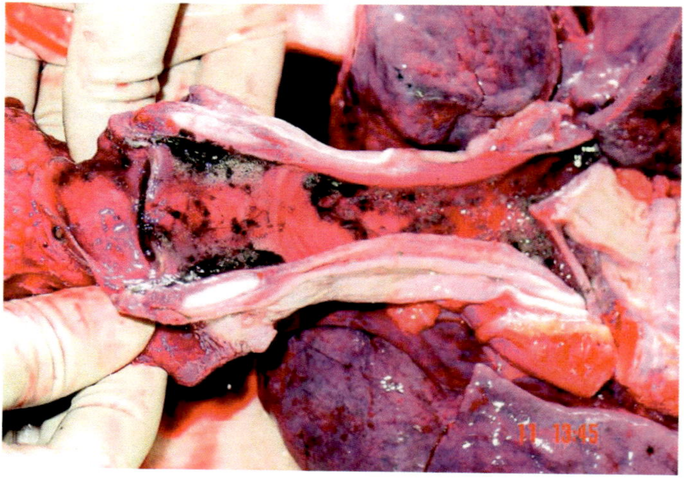

FIGURE 6.17: Presence of soot mixed with mucus in the respiratory tract is considered as a proof that the victim was alive in the fire. Note the red velvety mucosa of respiratory tract due to inhalation of hot fumes and gases.

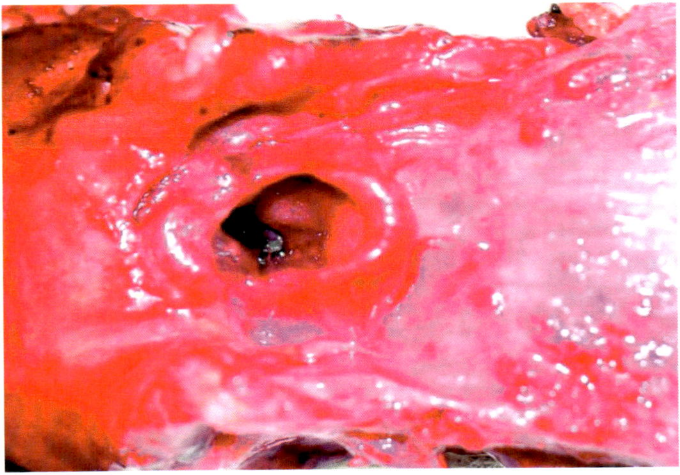

FIGURE 6.18: Edema of glottis, epiglottis and laryngeal mucosa can be noted if the victim had breathed the hot fumes and gases.

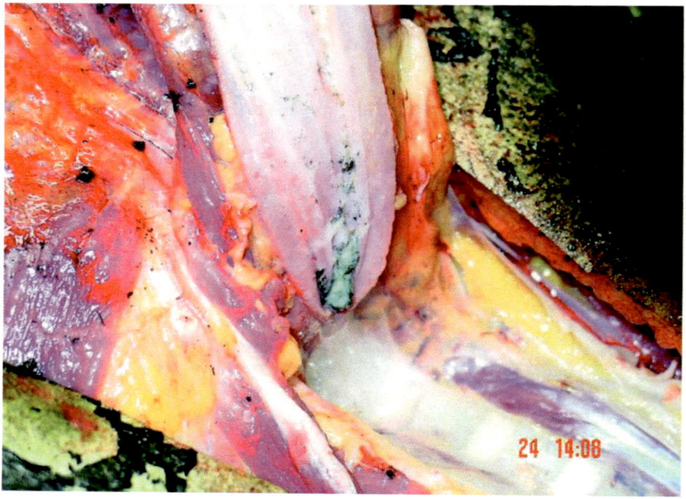

FIGURE 6.19: Presence of sputum mixed with soot in esophagus or stomach in a case of burn indicate that the victim was not only alive but had coughed inhaled soot and swallowed it.

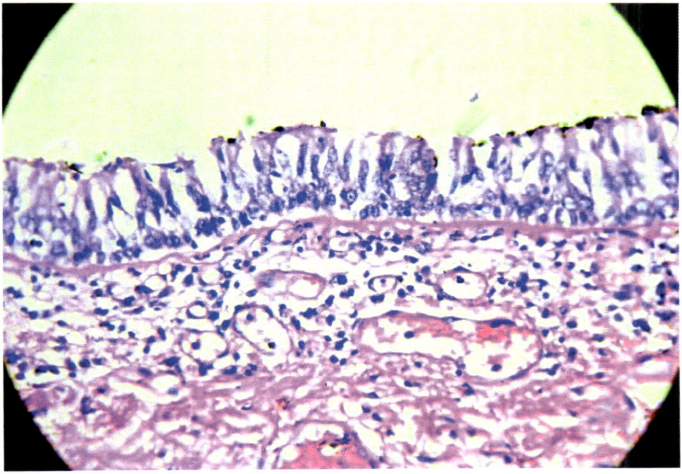

FIGURE 6.20: Soot particles lining the respiratory mucosa (X400 H and E stain).

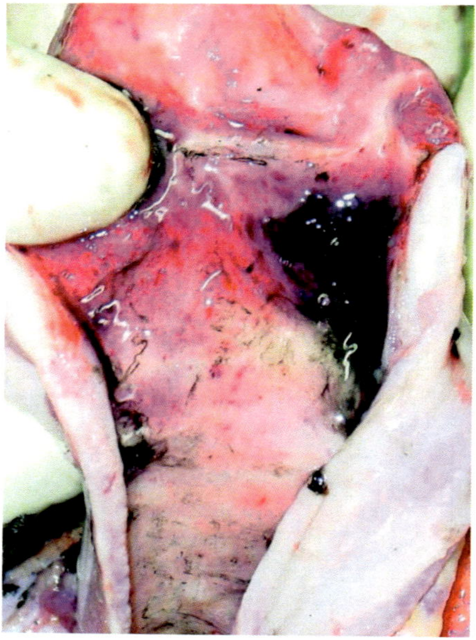

FIGURE 6.21: Submucosal petechial hemorrhages in the epiglottis, larynx and upper part of trachea may be found in the cases of burns.

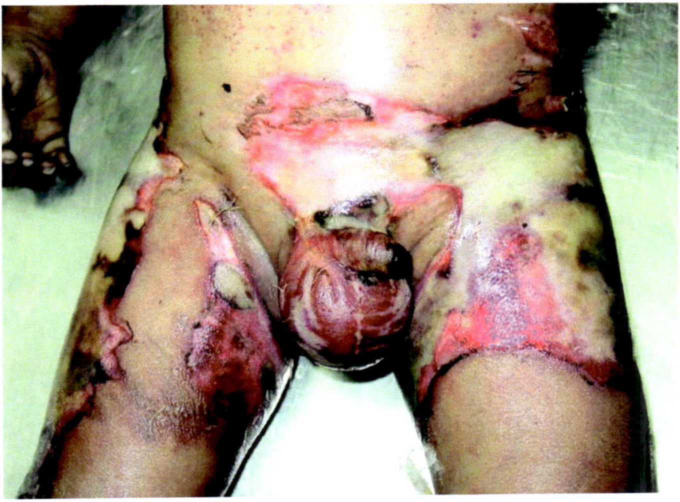

FIGURE 6.22: Scalds caused by hot water. Note that there is no blackening or soot. Hair is not burnt in the area of scald.

The immediate cause of death in cases of burn depends on the depth of burn, percentage of burnt body surface area and carboxyhemoglobin percentage of blood. Delayed deaths are usually caused by laryngeal edema, pulmonary edema, hypovolumic shock, consolidation of lungs, septicemia or gastrointestinal bleeding from its ulceration.

INJURIES CAUSED BY ELECTRICITY (FIGS 6.23 TO 6.27)

Injuries caused by electricity are known as electrocution injuries. The severity of electrocution injury depends on voltage (domestic supply of 220V at 50 Hz is fatal), type of current (alternating current is more dangerous than direct current), the resistance offered by the body (dry skin offers most resistance hence the skin is damaged due to electricity by heat formation at the site of contact to overcome the resistance) and the time period of contact of the electric conductor with the body surface. Death by electrocution is usually caused due to ventricular fibrillation or respiratory paralysis. Death by electrocution can be prevented by giving immediate resuscitative measures to the victim.

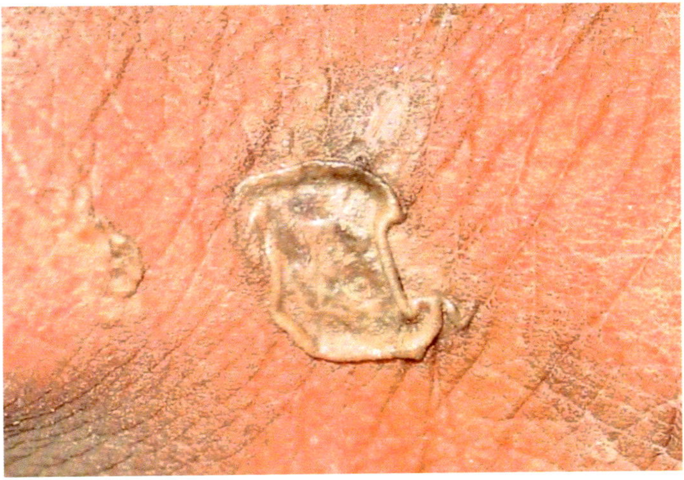

FIGURE 6.23: The typical entry wound of electrocution is rounded, hard, pale, sometimes black burnt tissue at the center, everted margin with zone of pale skin followed by zone of hyperemia. The zone of hyperemia disappears with passing time after death. As the electric current comes in contact with dry skin, the skin offers resistance. To overcome this resistance there is heat formation at the site of contact. Burn injury to skin produces a vesicle. However further contact with heat evaporates the fluid in the vesicle and desiccate or completely burn the skin which produces this appearance. No or very less damage can be seen if the skin coming in contact with electric conductor is wet or moist.

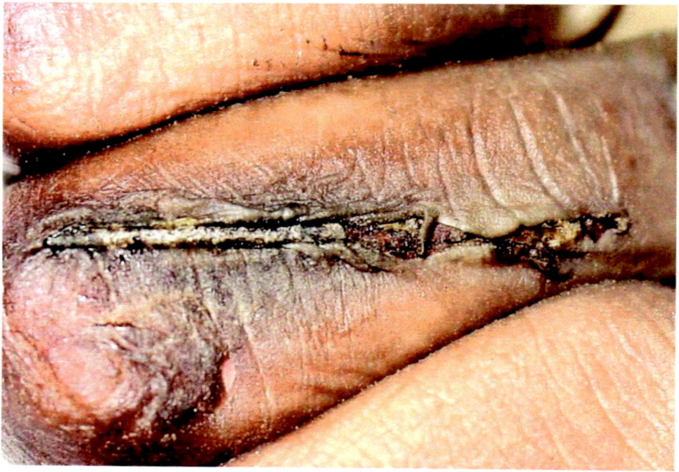

FIGURE 6.24: Sometimes the entry wound depicts the shape of electric conductor.

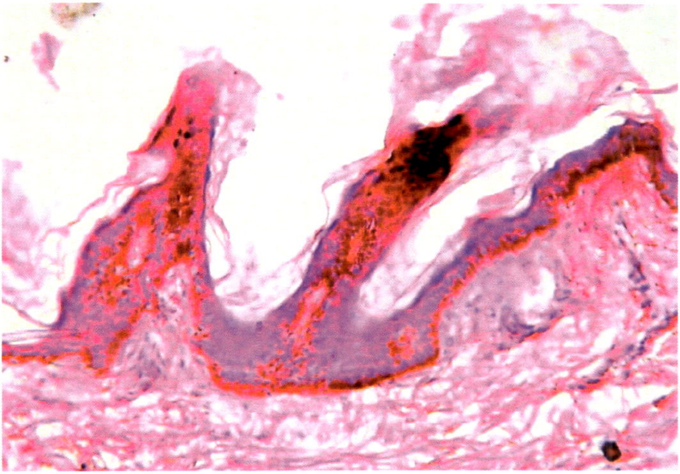

FIGURE 6.25: Histology of electrocution shows the findings consistent with that of injuries caused by heat (X100 H and E stain).

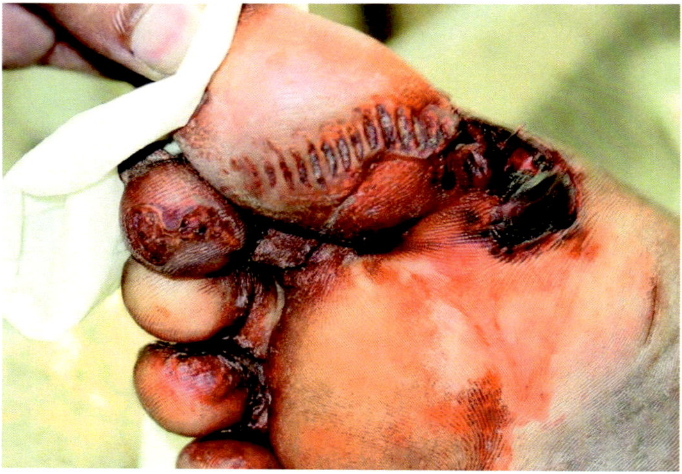

FIGURE 6.26: Sometimes an exit wound of electrocution can be seen. Here it has depicted the print caused by metal spring in contact with the foot.

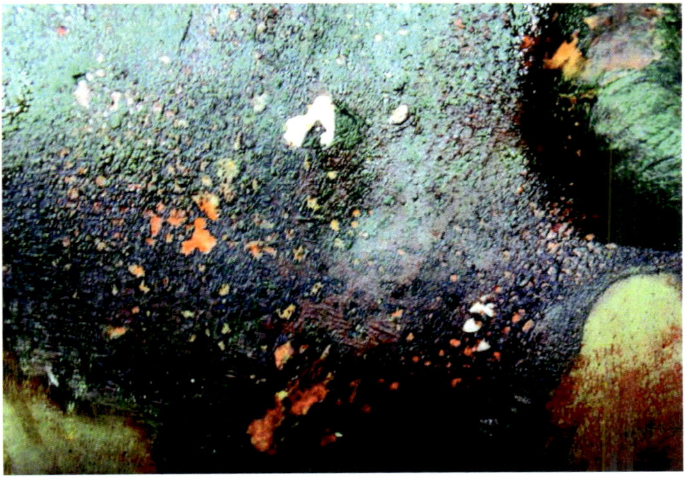

FIGURE 6.27: Severe burns may be caused by flash of high voltage current directly over body surface.

Internally no specific findings can be detected. Skin from the entry wound should be sent to forensic science lab for metal elements detection.

INJURIES CAUSED BY LIGHTNING (FIGS 6.28 TO 6.33)

History of thunderstorm is a very important piece of information as in many cases of death from lightning there is no injury or damage to the body. These deaths are purely accidental. Damage to the victim may be found when the victim is directly struck by lightning. The damage occurs due to very high voltage electricity, heat and blast effect of the expanding air column.

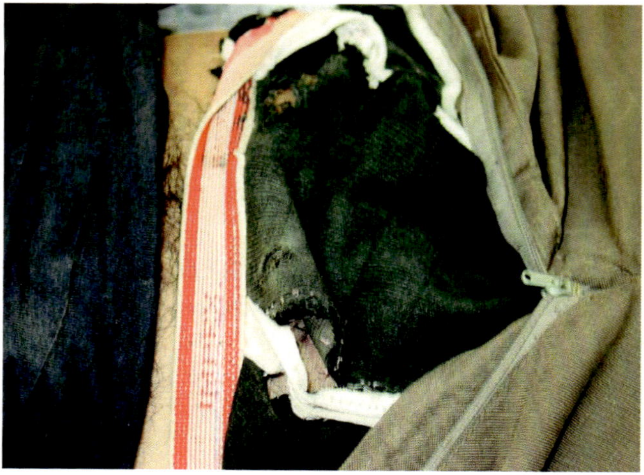

FIGURE 6.28: The clothes are torn at places due to blast effect. The elastic material in clothes like underpants may be found melted due to heat.

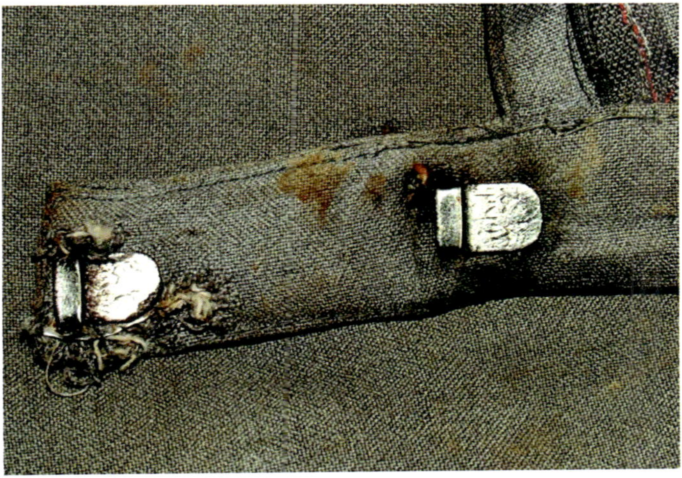

FIGURE 6.29: Blackening and scorching of clothes can be seen due to heating of the metal articles which come in contact with the clothes. In this case it is seen around the buckles of trousers. The metal articles may turn into magnet due to passing of electricity through it. However it may be lost due to heat or blast effect.

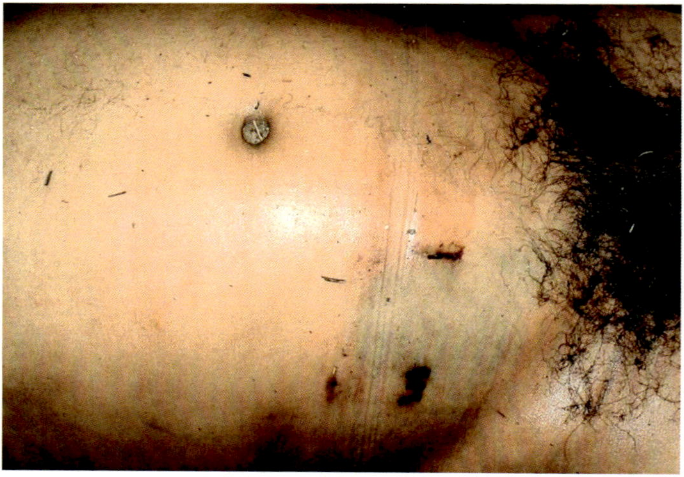

FIGURE 6.30: The body surface which is in contact with metallic objects may show burn injuries. Here in this case the burns are caused by metal buckles of trousers.

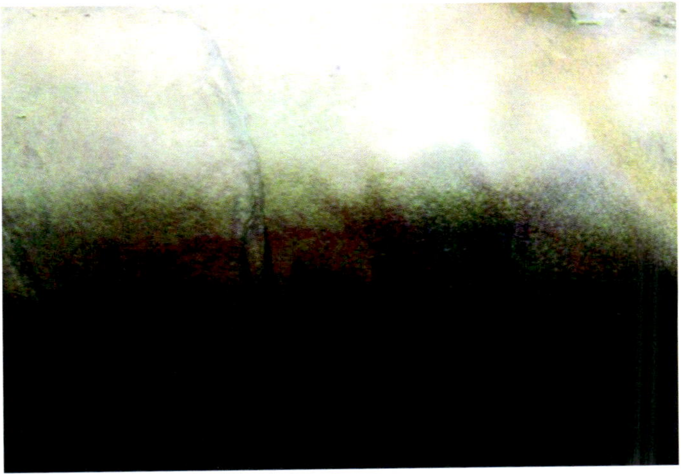

FIGURE 6.31: Filigree burns are not commonly seen. However if they are present, they are considered as a cardinal sign of lightning strike.

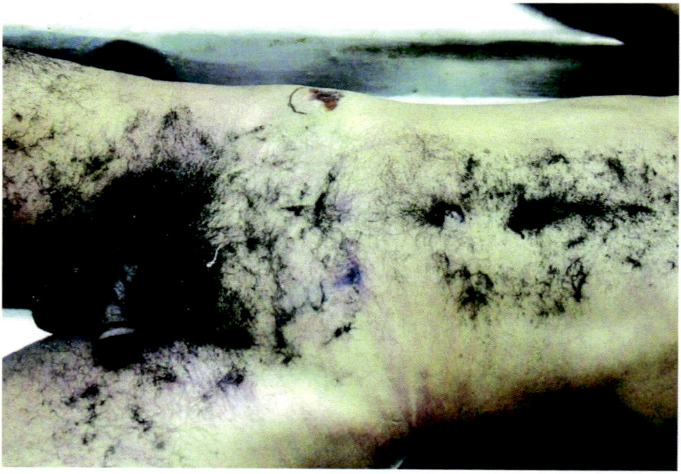

FIGURE 6.32: Singeing of body hair can be seen in the path of lightning over the body without any burns of overlying clothing.

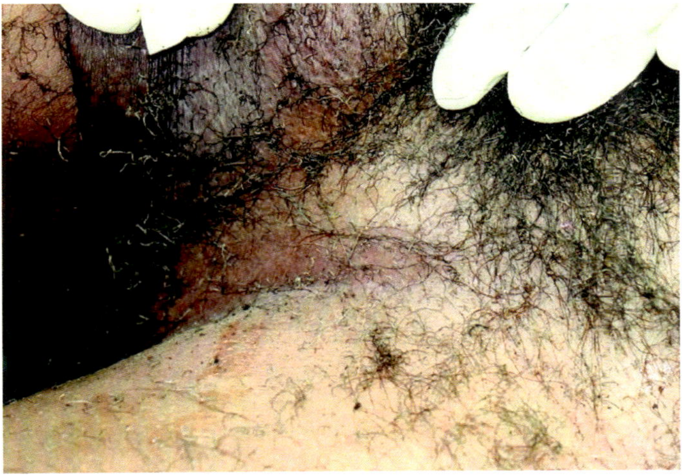

FIGURE 6.33: Heat wave passing over the body cause the moisture or sweat in the body creases to evaporate which produces superficial burns in these creases. (Note in burns caused by flames the skin in the creases is usually spared).

Death in the cases of lightning is usually caused by cardiac standstill. Immediate resuscitation is a great help to save the life of victim. A non-reacting pupil to light is no criteria for brain death in these cases. There are cases on record in which the victim of lightning survived when he was resuscitated after fifteen minutes following the lightning strike. Internally no specific findings can be detected other than non-specific petechial hemorrhages on the organs.

7 Mechanical Asphyxia and Drowning

Asphyxia means complete or partial lack of oxygen supply. It can be classified as mechanical asphyxia when it is caused due to mechanical blockage of respiratory tract, e.g. smothering, hanging, traumatic asphyxia, etc. and non-mechanical asphyxia when it is caused by causes other than mechanical asphyxia, e.g. poisoning, lung disease, etc.

SIGNS OF ASPHYXIA (FIGS 7.1 TO 7.7)

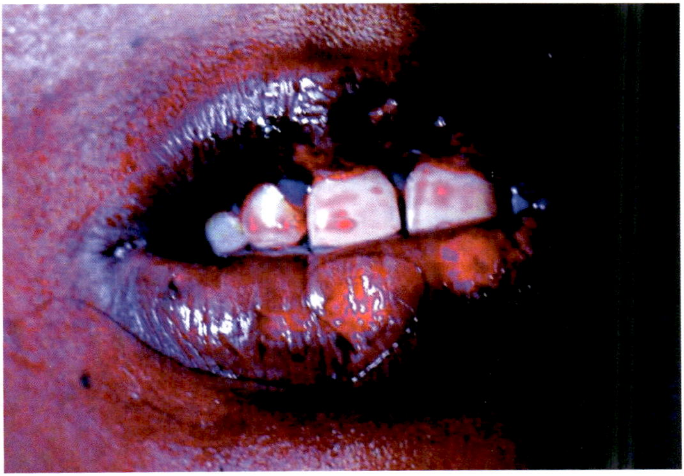

FIGURE 7.1: Cyanosis is violet discoloration of skin, nails, lips and ear lobules. It occurs when concentration of reduced hemoglobin in the blood reaches to 5 mg/100 cc of capillary blood. Internally it can be noticed as dark violet discoloration of organs. In this photograph cyanosis can be seen over lips as well as gums. Aquatic animal bites are present over lips.

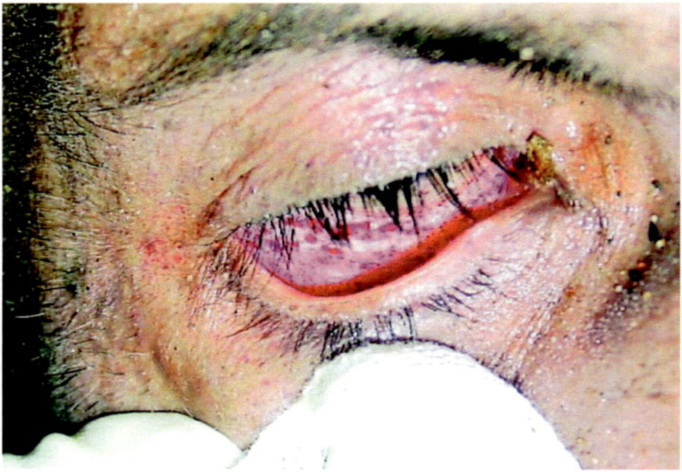

FIGURE 7.2: Petechial hemorrhages in the skin and palpebral conjunctiva are considered a sign of asphyxia.

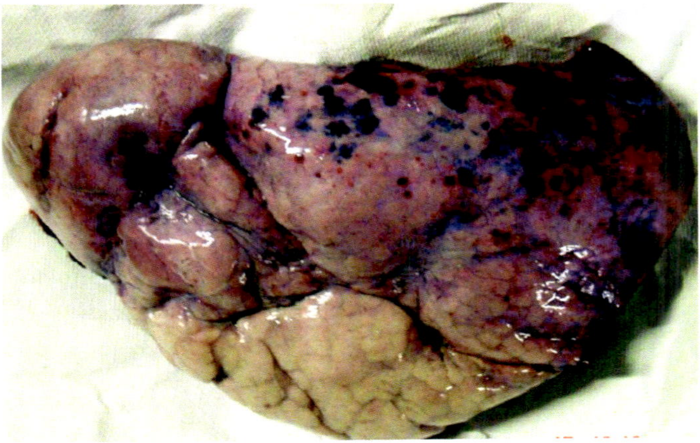

FIGURE 7.3: Petechial hemorrhages over organs are also considered a sign of asphyxia. This photograph shows petechi in lung.

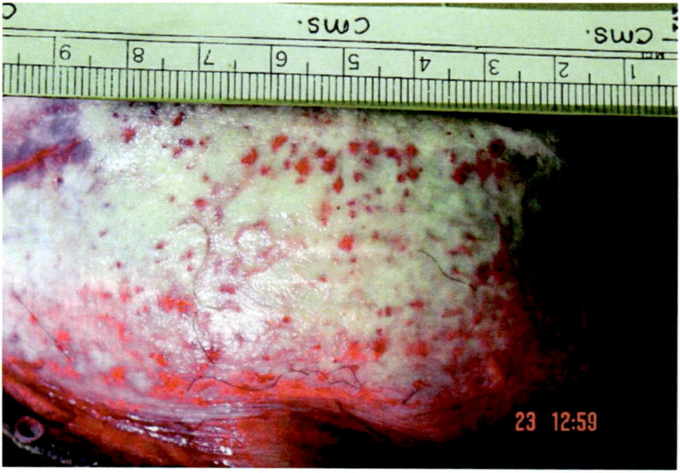

FIGURE 7.4: Petechial hemorrhages under scalp can be seen frequently in asphyxial death.

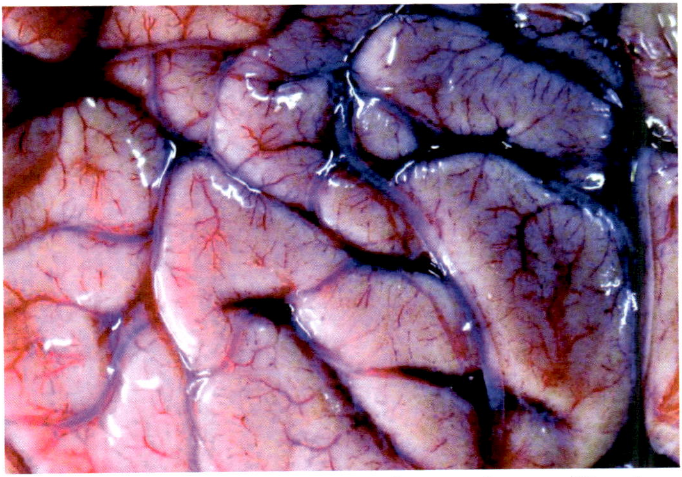

FIGURE 7.5: Congestion of face and organs is one of the signs of asphyxia. This photograph shows congested brain with air-bubbles in arteries as postmortem artifact.

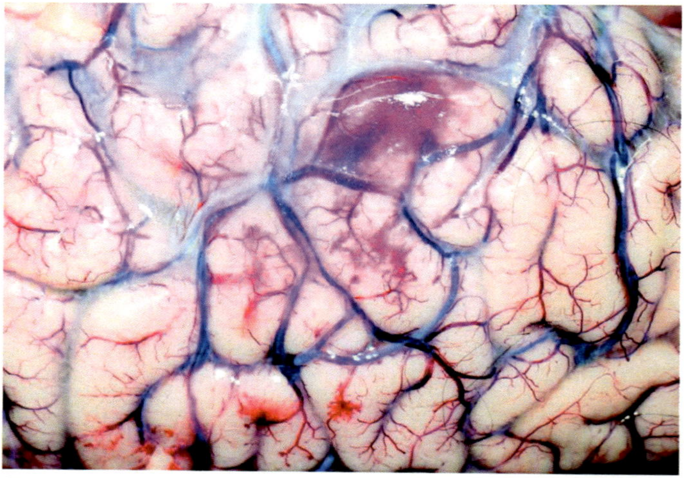

FIGURE 7.6: Focal subarachnoid hemorrhages are commonly seen in asphyxial deaths.

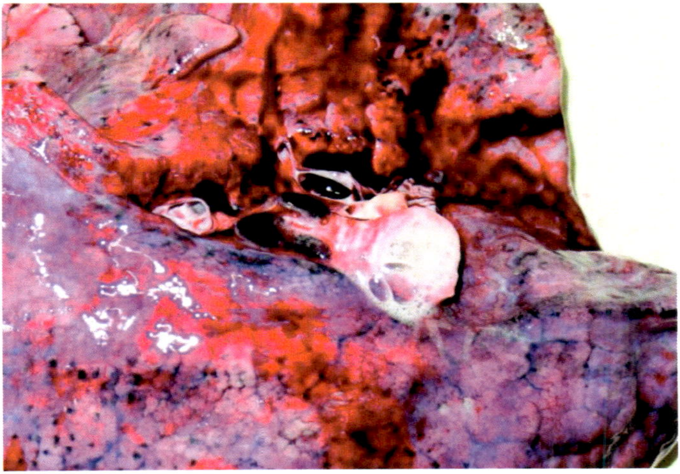

FIGURE 7.7: Pulmonary edema and edema of other organs are also common findings in asphyxial death.

Other finding includes persistent postmortem fluidity and dark red color of blood.

Although there are many causes of each of these findings, asphyxia can be considered as mode of death when maximum of the enumerated findings are present in a dead body. It must be remembered that in many occasions the mode of death is not asphyxia in so called "violent asphyxial deaths".

HANGING (FIGS 7.8 TO 7.23)

It is a form of death where the body is suspended partially or completely by applying ligature material around neck and constricting force being weight of body or partial weight of body.

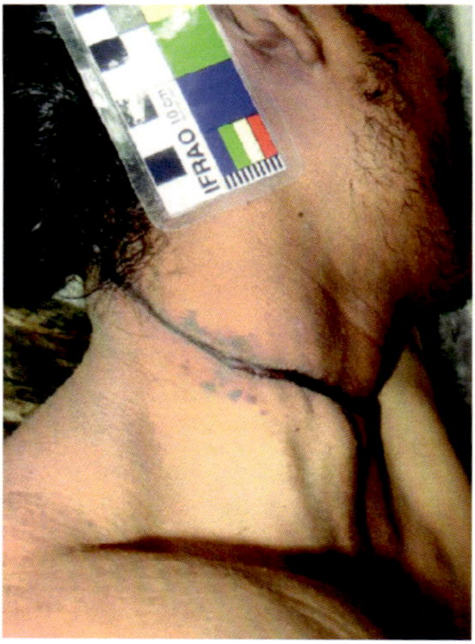

FIGURE 7.8: Partial or complete suspension of the body cause obliquely placed ligature mark irrespective of its position around thyroid cartilage. Different types of lesions can be found around the ligature mark. In this case multiple ecchymotic areas are present below and above ligature mark. When they are present above the ligature mark possibility of their postmortem appearance cannot be denied. However, when they are present below ligature mark they are invariably antemortem in nature.

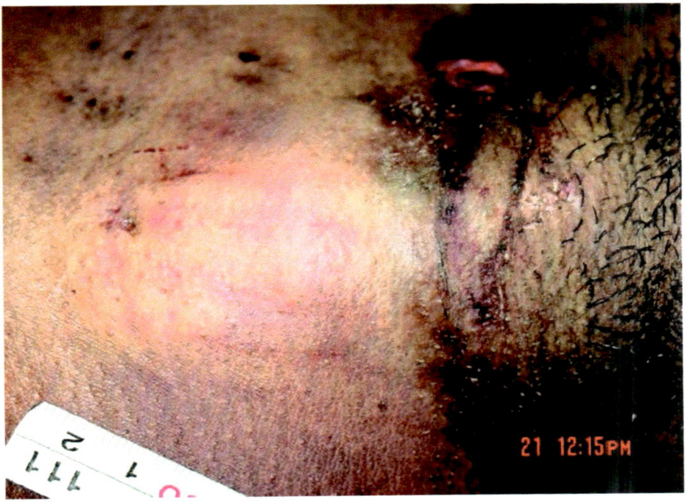

FIGURE 7.9: In hanging, when the loop gets pulled upwards due to weight of body below the neck, sometimes it causes abrasions directed upwards towards ligature mark known as the 'evidence of slippage of ligature material', which is considered sign of antemortem hanging.

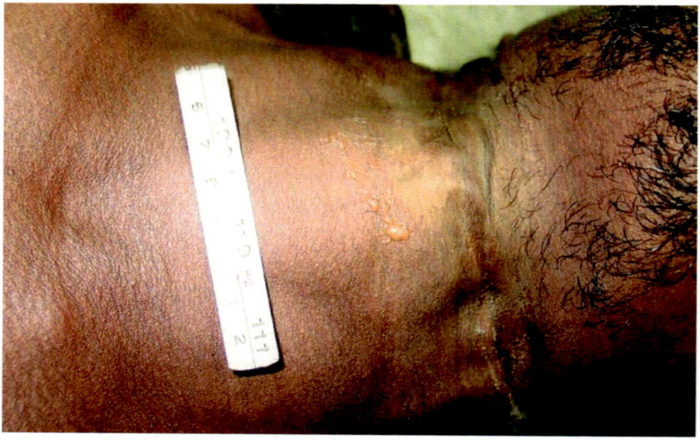

FIGURE 7.10: There may be vesiculation due to friction of ligature material with skin. Usually such vesicles are found at the margin of the ligature mark. Vesicles may be found in the skin squeezed between two winds of ligature material. In this case lungee (a cloth worn by males, wrapped around the waist to cover the waist and lower limbs) was used as a ligature material.

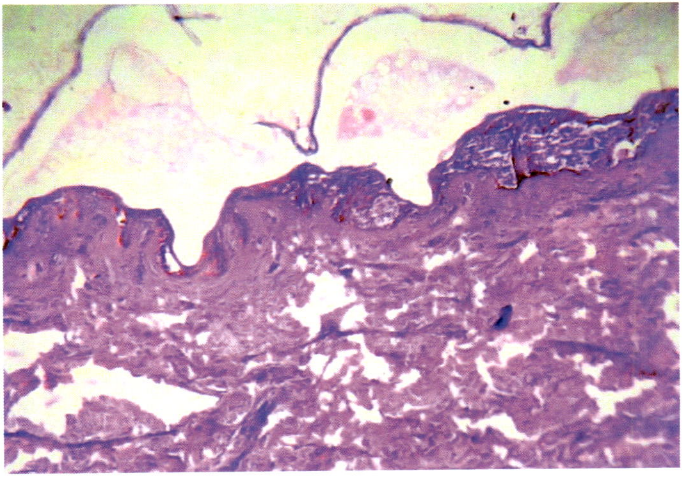

FIGURE 7.11: Whether these vesicles are antemortem or postmortem is to be decided after histological study of the lesion. As in this case, there is presence of protein contained fluid, indicating its antemortem origin (X100 H and E stain).

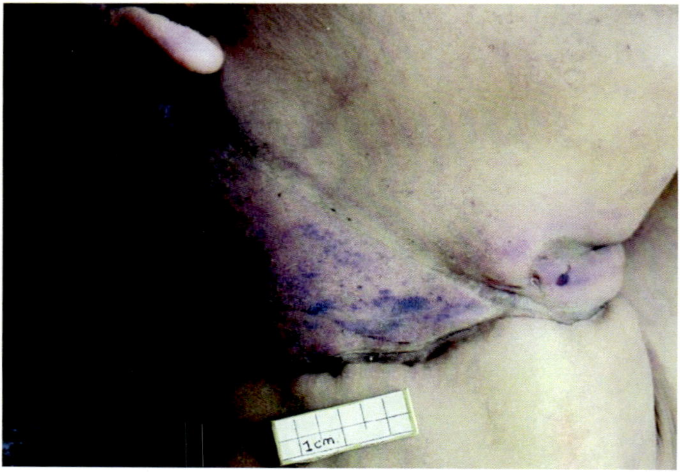

FIGURE 7.12: When the broad area of skin gets squeezed between two winds of ligature mark then it may show congestion, petechiae or ecchymotic patches. Whether they are antemortem or postmortem in origin is to be decided after histological study as their postmortem origin can not be denied.

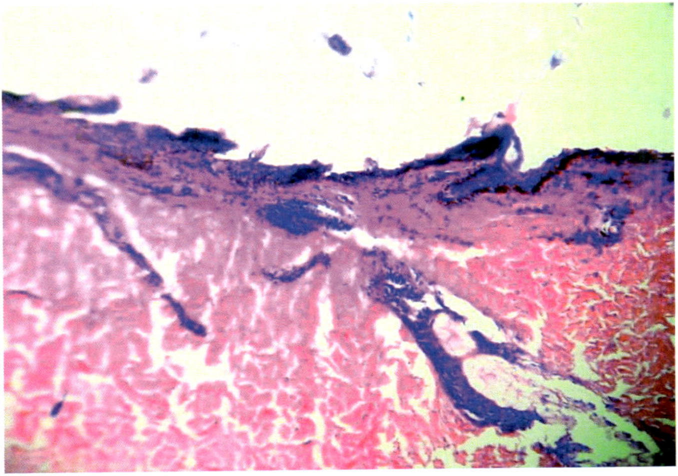

FIGURE 7.13: Frequently the histological study of ligature mark reveals features of abrasion without any extravasation of blood in the dermis or subcutaneous tissue. Hence it is very difficult to decide whether the mark is antemortem or postmortem (X100 H and E stain).

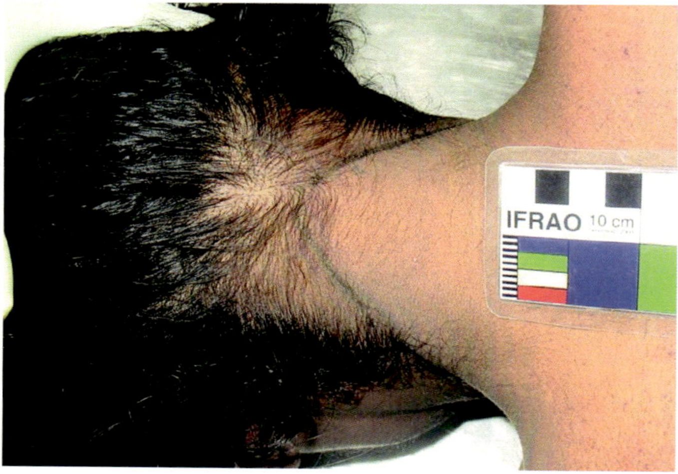

FIGURE 7.14: When the obliquely running ligature mark ends on occiput or back of neck then it is a case of typical hanging. It is usually absent at its upper point.

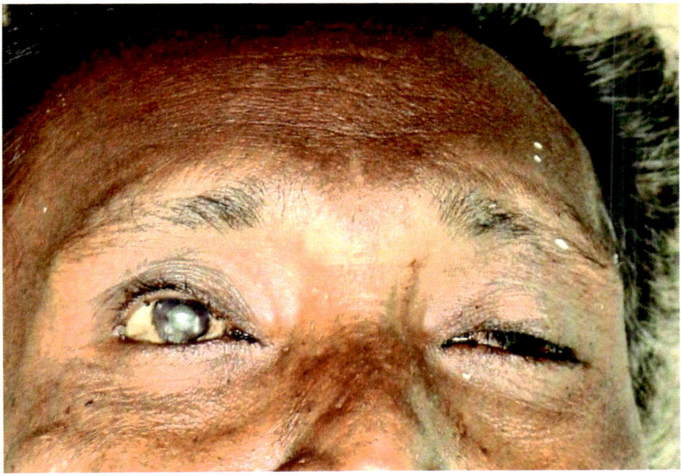

FIGURE 7.15: "Le facie sympathique" considered as a sign of antemortem hanging. It is due to compression of ligature material on cervical sympathetic, the eye on the same side may remain open and its pupil dilated indicating antemortem hanging.

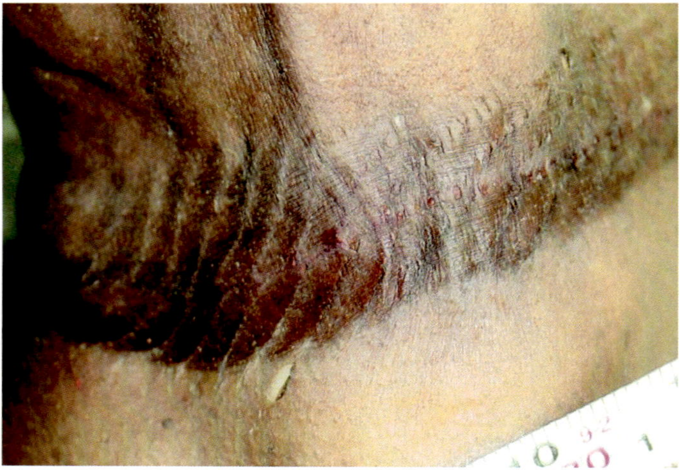

FIGURE 7.16: The ligature mark may depict the design of rope. Note tiny vesicles in the ligature mark.

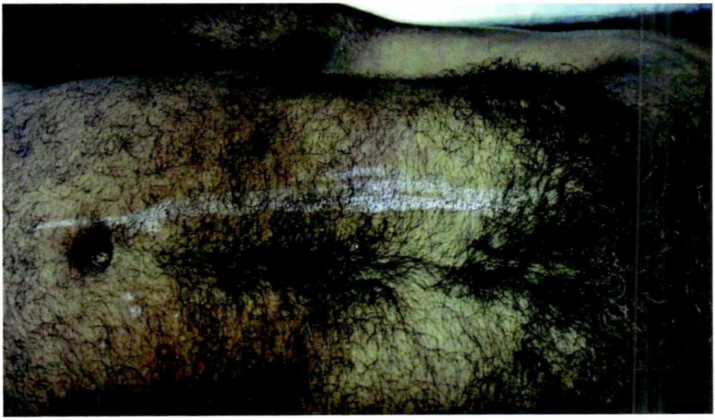

FIGURE 7.17: Dribbled saliva is considered as an evidence of antemortem hanging. However, this stain may be lost, if the body is kept in cold storage and condensation occurs on body surface after taking it out prior to autopsy.

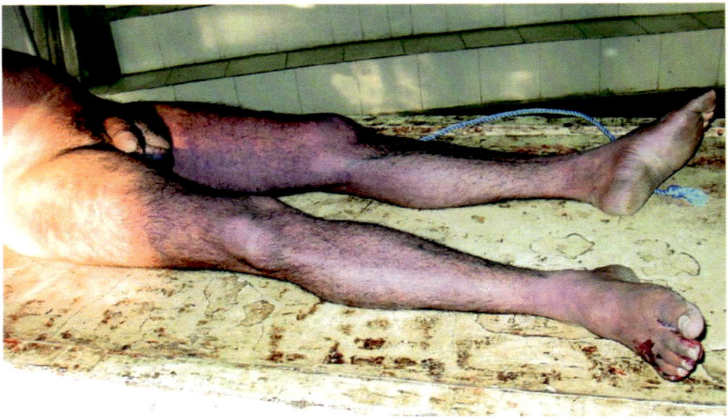

FIGURE 7.18: Gloves and stocking type of postmortem lividity is evident if the body is suspended for more than about six hours.

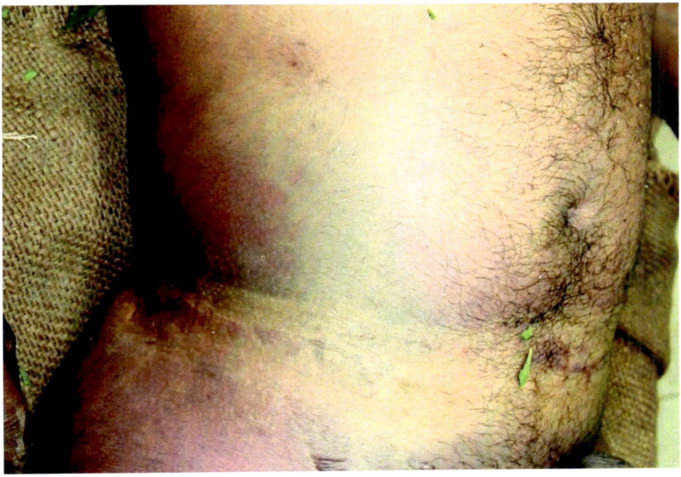

FIGURE 7.19: The postmortem lividity appears above the clothes tied around waist.

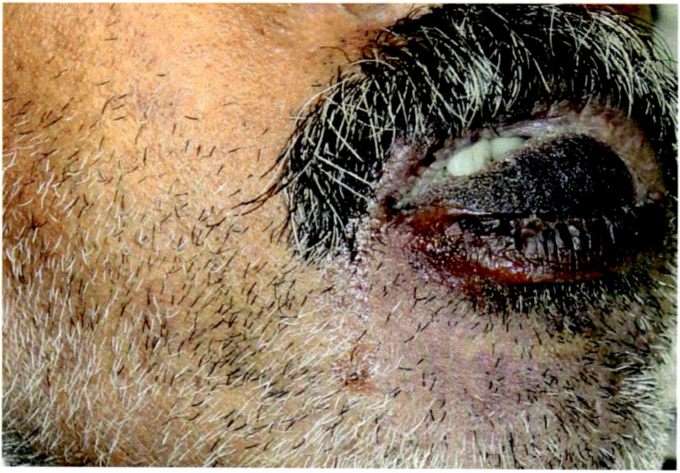

FIGURE 7.20: Protrusion of tongue is commonly present in hanging but it is not a proof of hanging as it may be found in many other deaths as agonal changes.

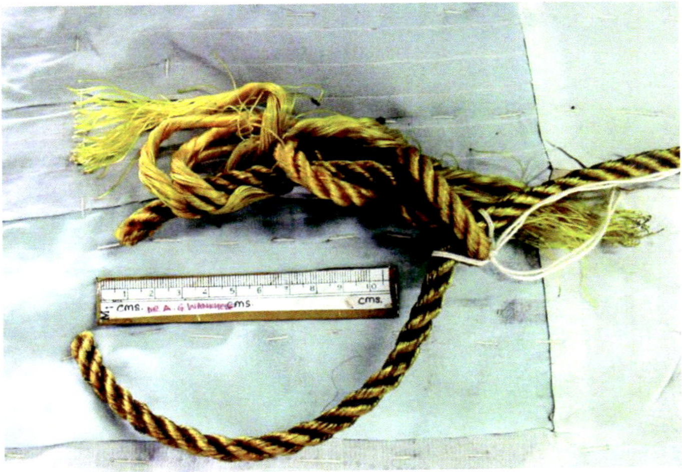

FIGURE 7.21: Ligature material if present *in situ* should be removed by cutting opposite to the knot to preserve it. While measuring the length of ligature materials it must be mentioned whether the length is measured while the material was stretched or unstretched.

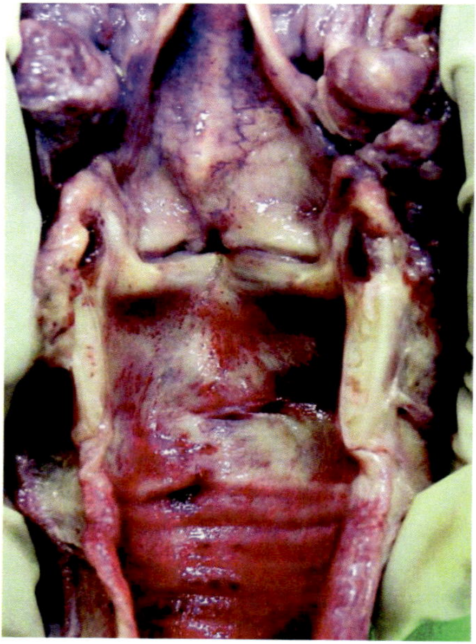

FIGURE 7.22: There may not be any internal damage in the neck structures due to hanging. Fracture of hyoid bone and thyroid cartilage if present are with either minimal or no extravasation of blood. The maximum possible findings are submucosal petechial hemorrhages in base of tongue, epiglottis, pharynx and larynx. As in this case it can be seen that the cricoid cartilage and first tracheal ring are fractured.

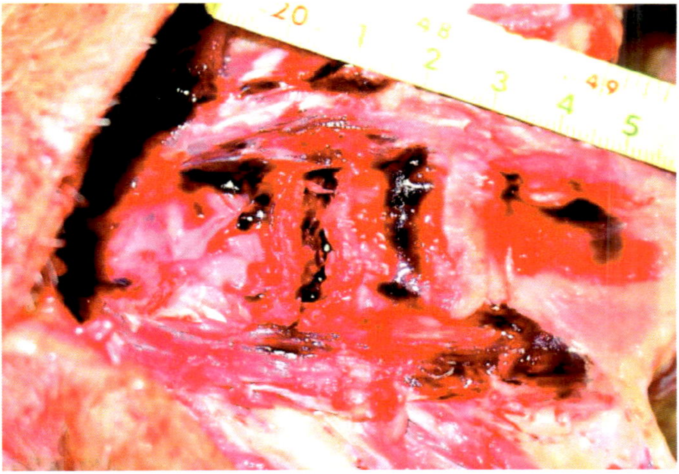

FIGURE 7.23: Hanging with long drop or jerk may cause fracture dislocation of cervical spine and damages to spinal cord.

STRANGULATION (FIGS 7.24 TO 7.32)

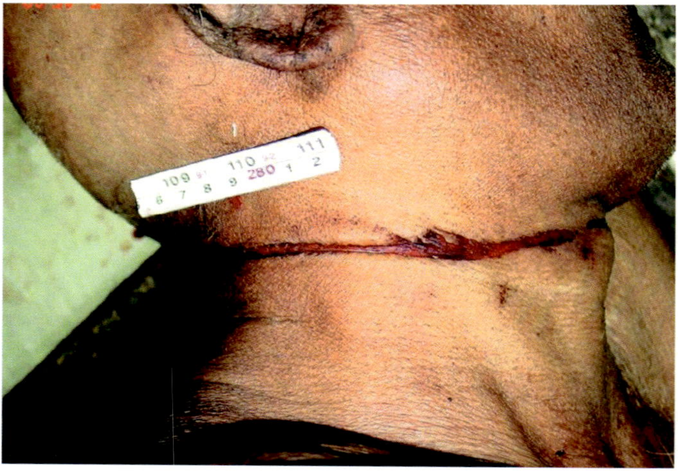

FIGURE 7.24: In ligature strangulation the ligature material is applied for constricting the neck without suspension of body and constricting force is other than the body weight. Hence the ligature mark is horizontal and continuous.

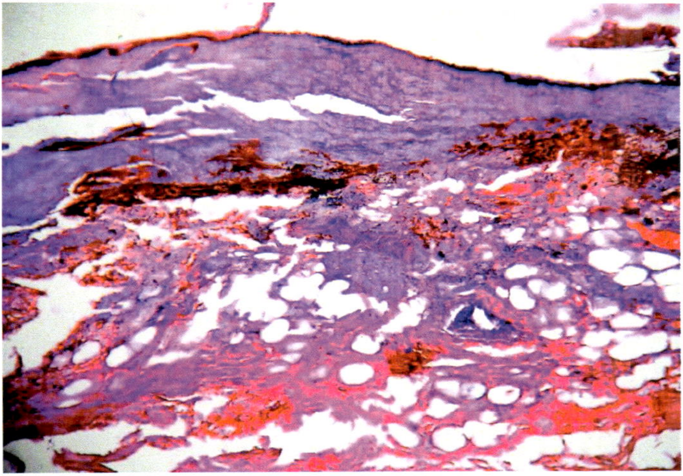

FIGURE 7.25: Histological study of ligature mark in strangulation frequently reveals extravasation of blood in the underlying dermis and subcutaneous tissue.

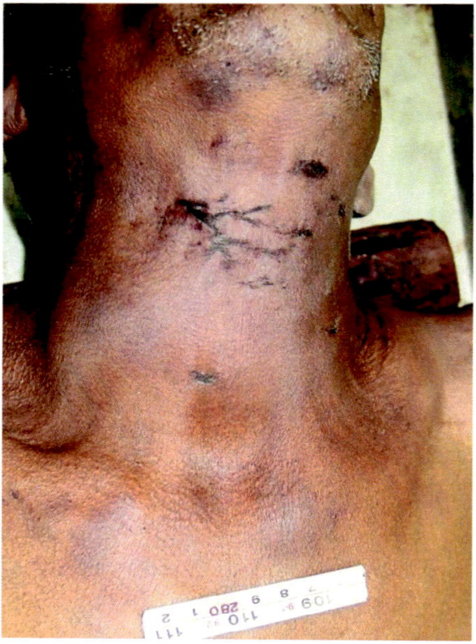

FIGURE 7.26: Manual strangulation or throttling is a form of death when the neck is constricted with the hands. Along with abrasions, huge bruises are very common in this type of strangulation.

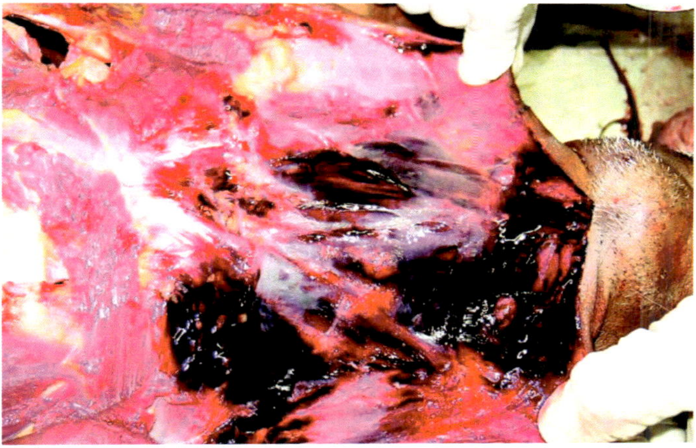

FIGURE 7.27: Internal damage is extensive in strangulation and throttling. Note the extravasated blood in muscles and soft tissue of neck.

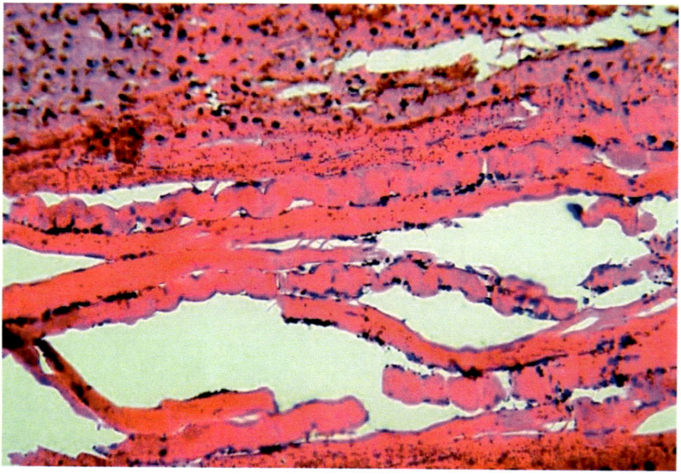

FIGURE 7.28: Histological study commonly reveals extravasation of blood in muscle tissue with injury to muscle fibers. Note the wavy muscle fibers (X400 H and E stain).

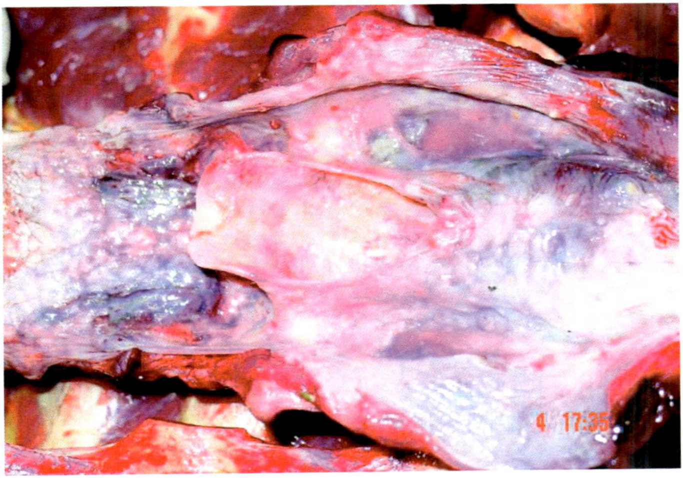

FIGURE 7.29: Submucosal hemorrhages in base of the tongue, pharynx, epiglottis, and glottis are very common in strangulation.

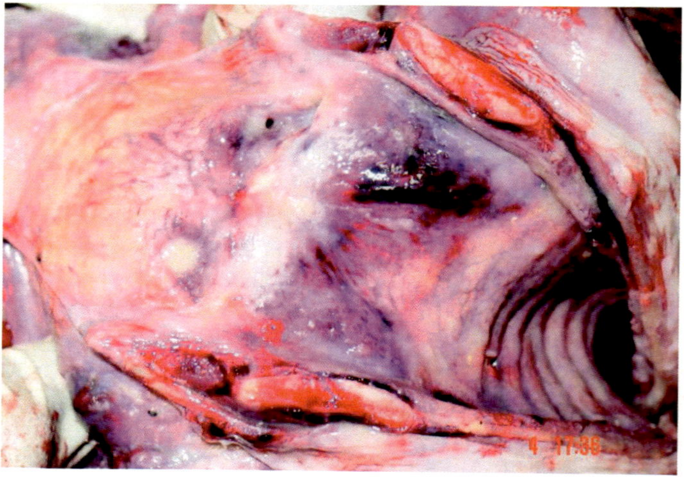

FIGURE 7.30: Laryngeal submucosal hemorrhages with fractures of laryngeal cartilages can be found in strangulation.

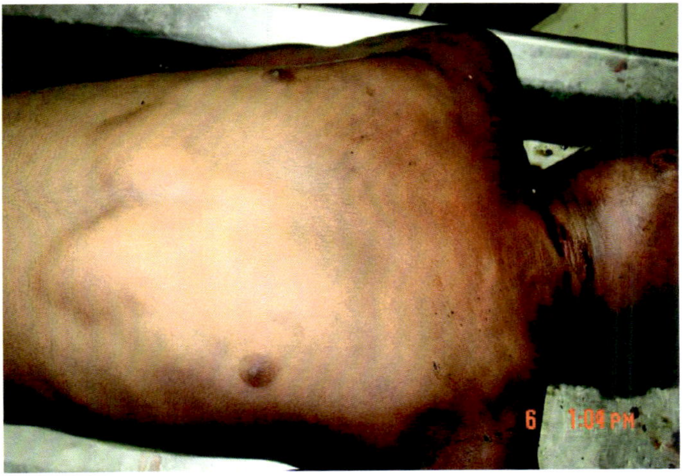

FIGURE 7.31: Accidental strangulation may cause laceration of larynx or trachea giving rise to emphysema in the soft tissue of neck and chest.

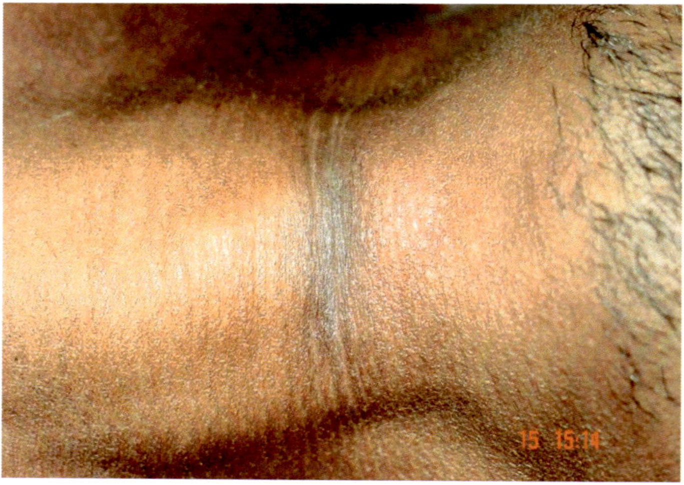

FIGURE 7.32: Sometimes neck creases may look like ligature marks. This phenomenon is quite common in decomposed bodies.

Other injuries due to struggle may be found on the deceased. The fibers, visible or microscopic, must be collected by lifting them by adhesive transparent tape and sticking it on glass slide in every case of ligature strangulation. They should be sent to forensic science lab with suspected ligature material and victim's clothes as a control sample.

Other mechanical asphyxial deaths include gagging (putting a gag into the mouth so that it causes blockage of respiratory tract at pharynx), smothering (the mouth and nostrils are blocked externally), traumatic asphyxia (the chest and abdominal walls are fixed), choking (respiratory tract blocked by a foreign body), plastic bag suffocation (when plastic bag is tied around face) and postural asphyxia (when the person died in head low position). In all these instances of mechanical asphyxia, signs of asphyxia are commonly well marked.

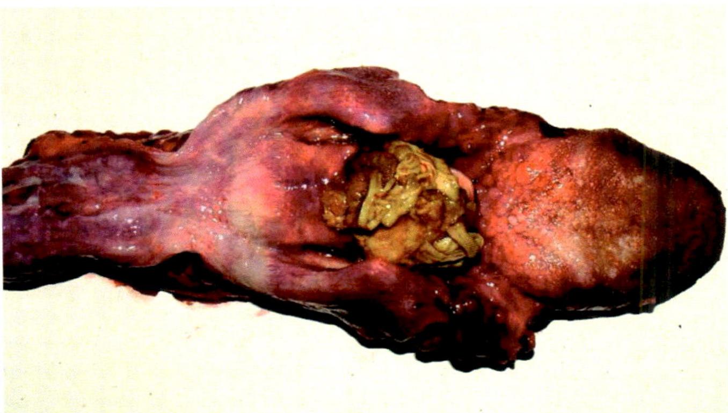

FIGURE 7.33: Choking is frequently seen in old people, children, alcoholic or psychiatric patients. However normal adult humans are not exceptions. Food material is the most common cause of choking. It is always surrounded by mucus secretions.

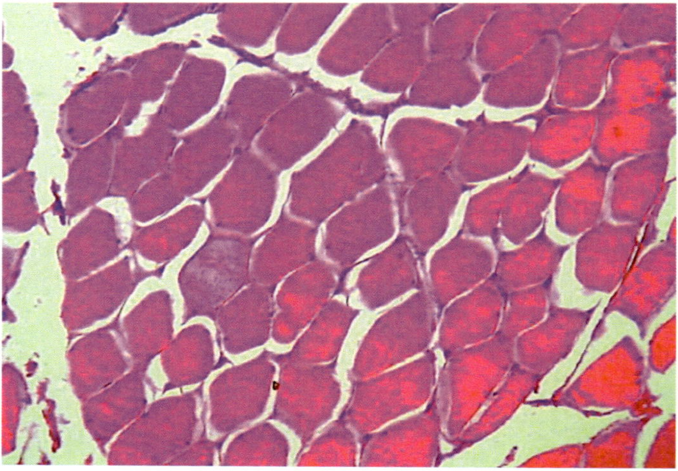

FIGURE 7.34: A Large piece of cooked meat is a common choking agent. However size of the bolus is not the criteria for choking. This is microscopic picture of cooked meat (X400 H and E stain).

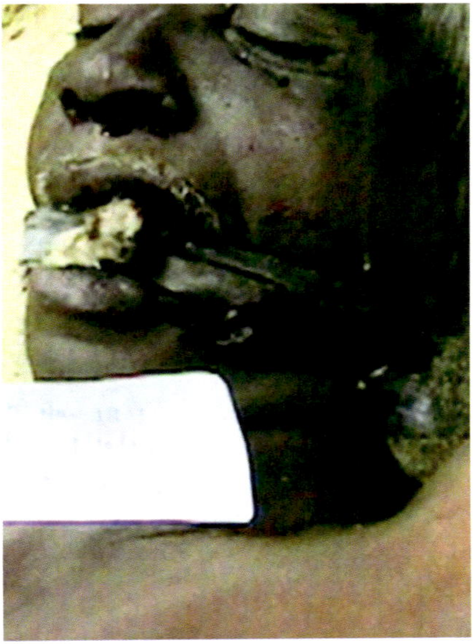

FIGURE 7.35: Death by gagging. (*Courtesy:* Dr Kailash U Zine, Associate Professor, Forensic Medicine, Govt. Medical College, Aurangabad).

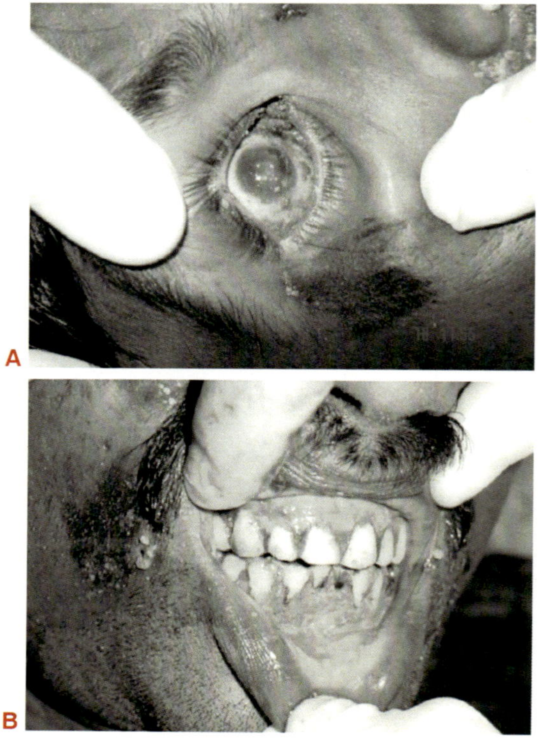

FIGURES 7.36A AND B: Death due to traumatic asphyxia associated with smothering as the victim gets trapped in the thick mud of his fallen hut. Note mud in his eyes and mouth. It was also present in his nostrils.

DROWNING (FIGS 7.37 TO 7.46)

It is a form of death in which air entry is blocked by entry of water in the respiratory tract due to submersion of face or body into water.

Postmortem findings in a case of drowning are due to:

A. Contact of body with water and (Figs 7.37 to 7.42)
B. Entry of water into respiratory tract (Figs 7.43 to 7.46)

Clothes are wet or moist. Mud, sand or aquatic weeds may be adherent to clothes. Sometimes aquatic animal may be found trapped in clothes.

FIGURE 7.37: Due to contact with cold water the skin becomes granular and puckered in appearance called as cutis anserina.

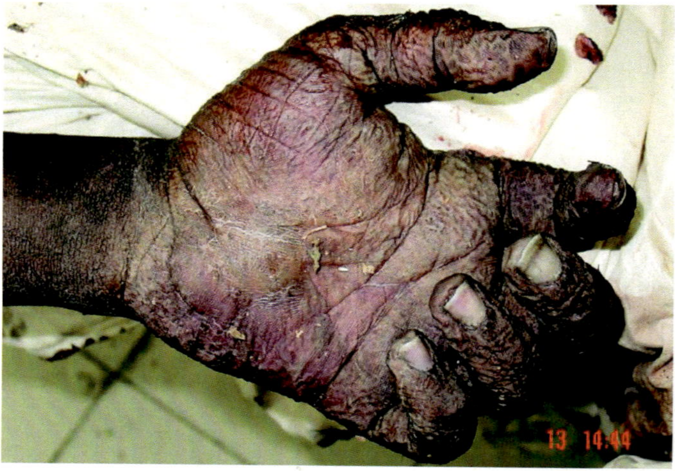

FIGURE 7.38: The skin becomes more and more white, sodden, wrinkled and thickened with increase in time of contact with water popularly called as sign of washer-woman's hands and feet. Note mud under the nails.

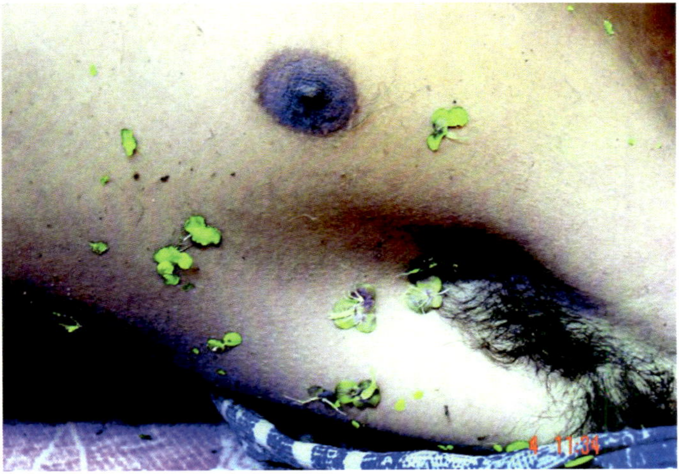

FIGURE 7.39: Aquatic weeds, mud or sand particles may be adherent to body surface.

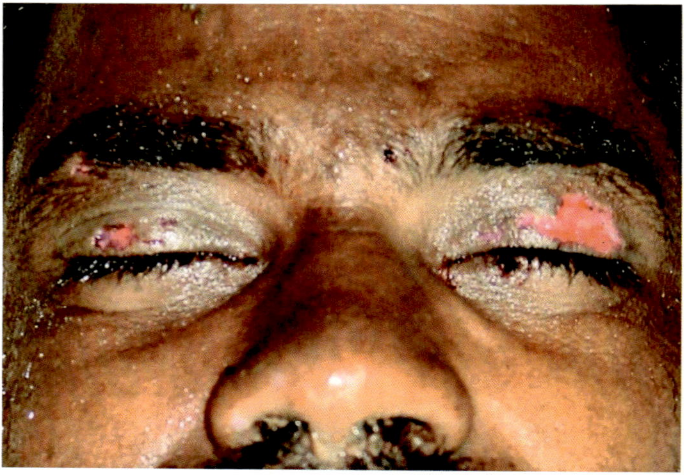

FIGURE 7.40: Aquatic animal bites can be seen on the soft parts of body.

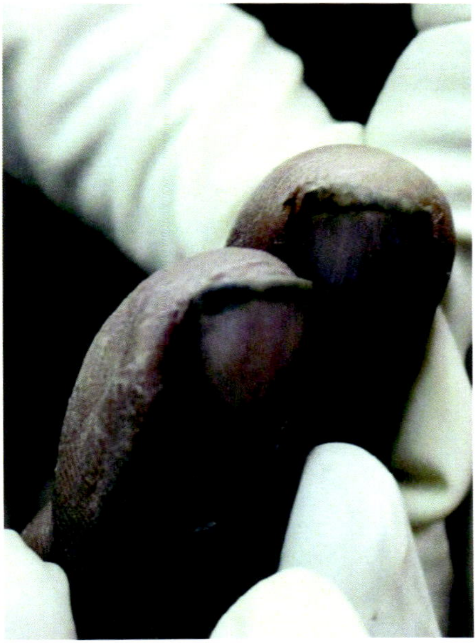

FIGURE 7.41: Mud or sand may be found under the nails of hands and it is considered as a sign of life while drowning as in the process of saving oneself the victim may grasp aquatic weeds (cadaveric spasm) or scratch over the water bed.

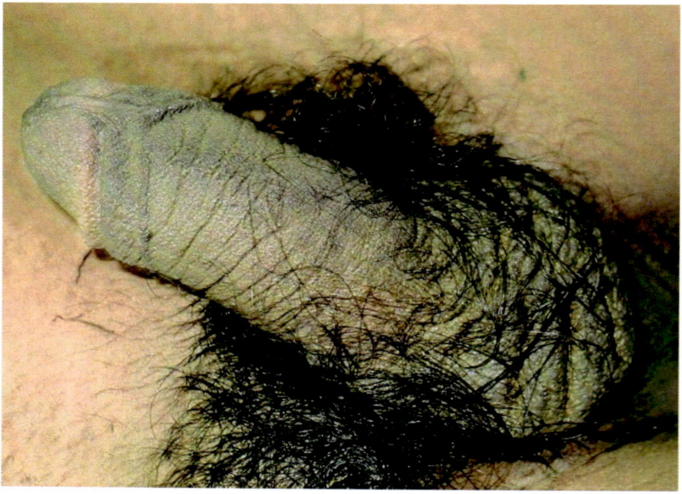

FIGURE 7.42: Scrotum and penis are retracted in body recovered from water.

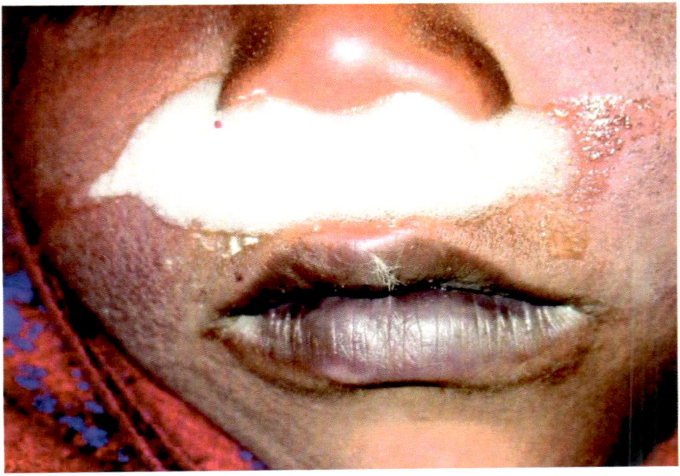

FIGURE 7.43: When the water enters into the respiratory tract either it causes laryngeal spasm followed by death or the respiratory tract tries to cough out the water and secretes mucus. However when water enters repeatedly, violent coughing causes churning of water, mucus and air giving rise to the typical white, fine, tenacious, lathery, copious and sometimes blood tinged froth which oozes from nostrils and mouth. This froth is diagnostic of drowning. Similar froth may be found in respiratory tract.

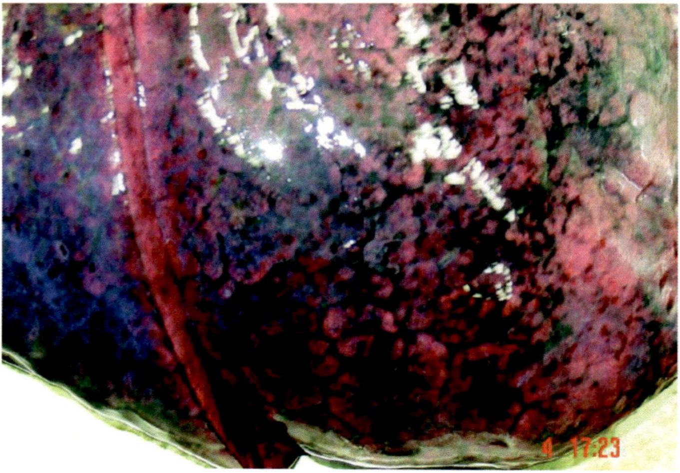

FIGURE 7.44: Lungs are usually voluminous, edematous and ballooning in cases of drowning. Paltauf's hemorrhages may be found on the surface of lung.

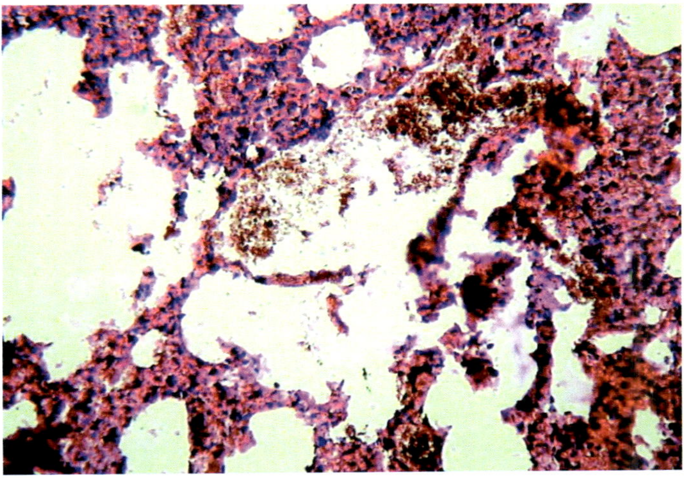

FIGURE 7.45: Paltauf's hemorrhages are caused by the rupture of alveolar wall due to sudden increase in pressure by forced expiration. This is considered as a sign of antemortem drowning (X100 H and E stain).

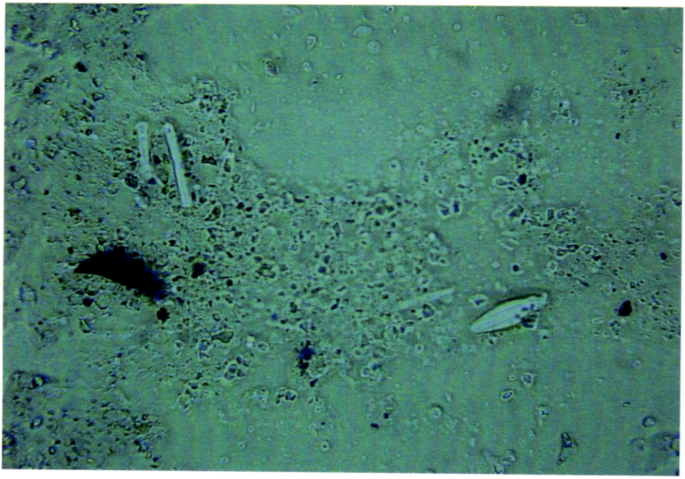

FIGURE 7.46: Diatoms from the water in which the victim succumbed can be found in the organs or bone marrow of the victim.

8 Starvation

Total deprivation of food causes starvation. The intake of food may be stopped suddenly or in a decreasing manner. Starvation is usually associated with neglect. The dead body of a starved victim usually emits a disagreeable odor. The clothes are absent or if present they are dirty.

GENERAL FINDINGS (FIGS 8.1 TO 8.7)

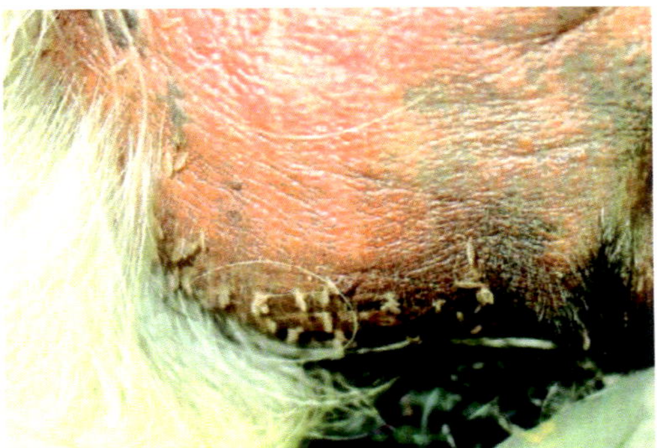

FIGURE 8.1: Insects like lice may be found in and around scalp hair.

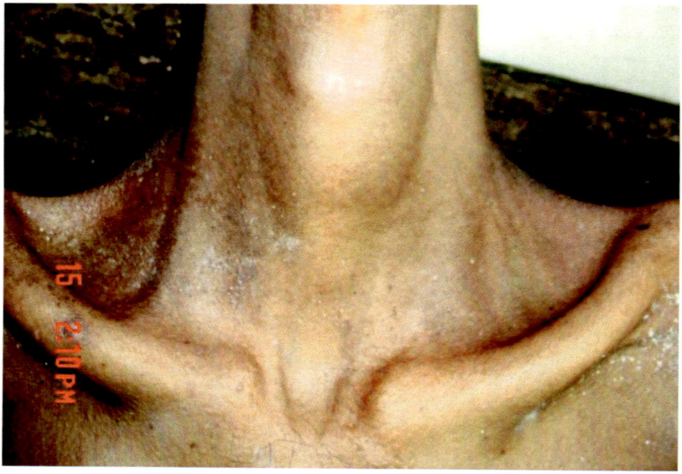

FIGURE 8.2: Complete loss of fat and muscle mass gives rise to emaciation of the victim. All bony areas become prominent.

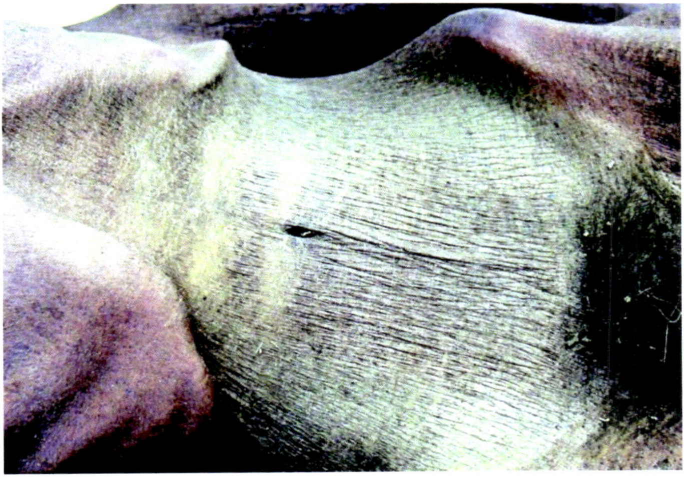

FIGURE 8.3: Abdomen of starved victim is concave (not scaphoid). However sometimes ascites may develop.

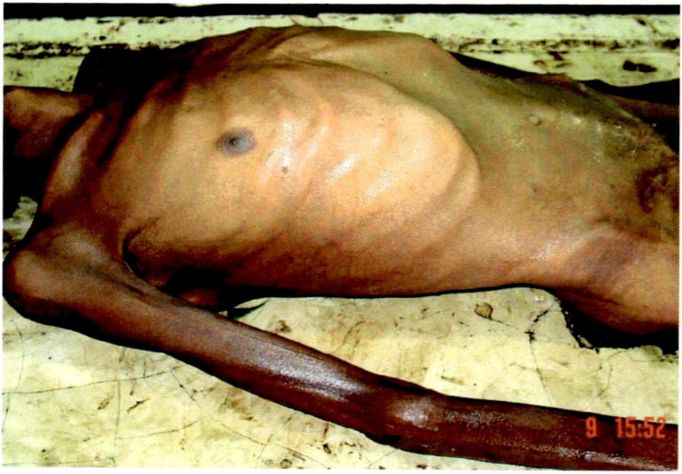

FIGURE 8.4: Both extremities become thin. Note slightly distended abdomen due to ascites.

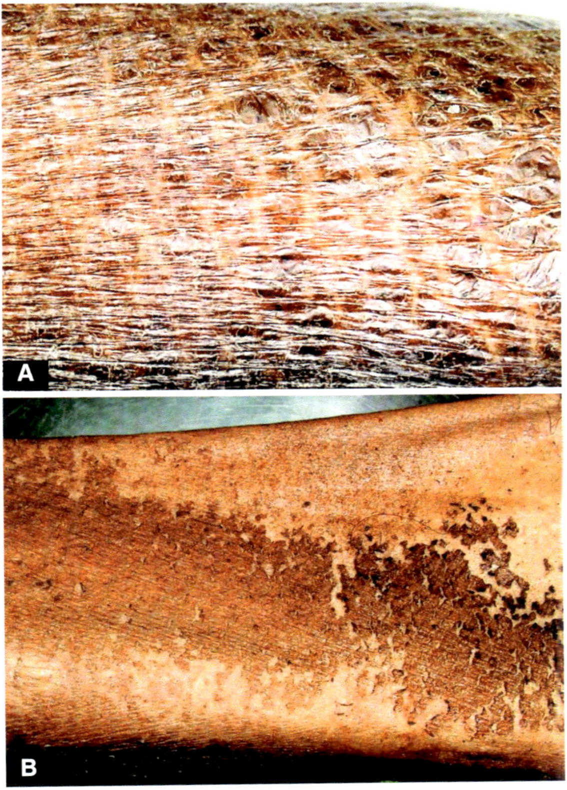

FIGURES 8.5A AND B: Skin is dry, dirty, cracked, and rough, emits beggary odor, inelastic, hyperpigmented and lanugo hair may be seen.

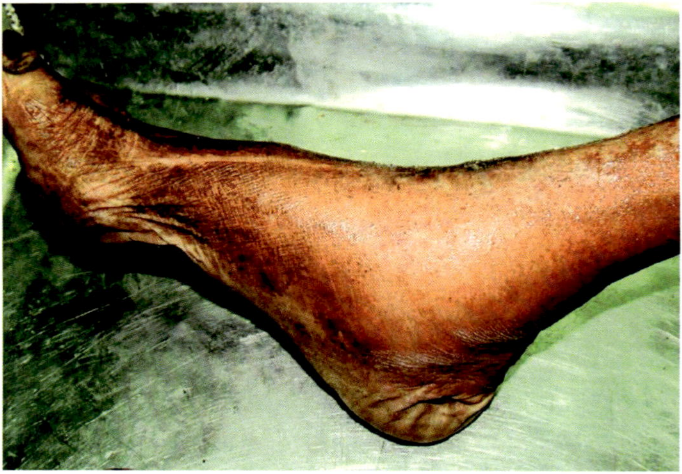

FIGURE 8.6: Infrequently joints are swollen.

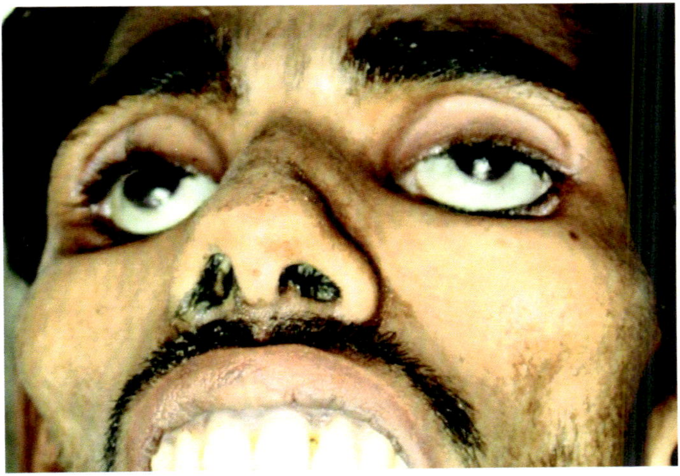

FIGURE 8.7: The eyes look sunken, white and glistening. Cheek bones become prominent due to loss of buccal fat.

INTERNAL FINDINGS (FIGS 8.8 TO 8.10)

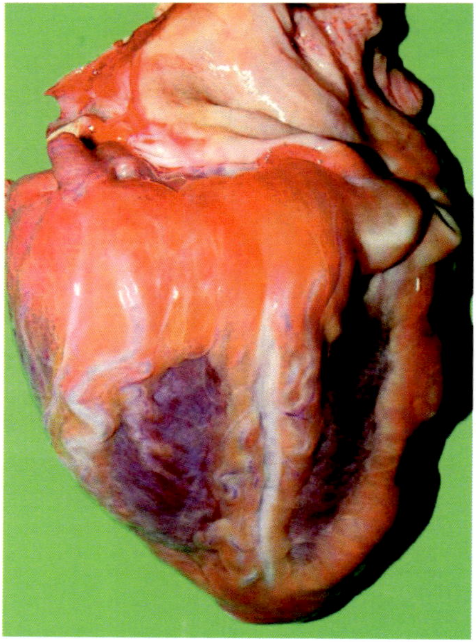

FIGURE 8.8: All organs except brain reduce in their size and weight. Infrequently multiple necrotic areas may be found in organs. Fat is present in only periorbital area and female breast. Epicardial fat is degenerated into a gelatinous mass.

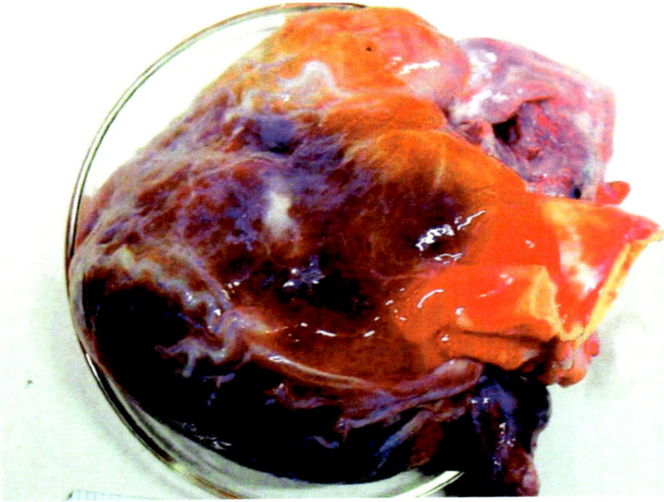

FIGURE 8.9: Sometimes this gelatinous mass may become watery.

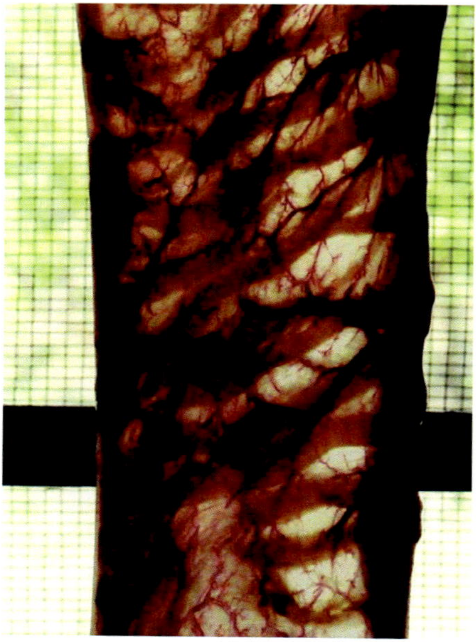

FIGURE 8.10: Stomach and intestine are empty or contains thick dark green bilious material. Walls of stomach and intestine become papery thin and translucent.

Chronic or old age diseases can be frequently found in the deceased of starvation.

9 Fetus

A baby from the eighth week of gestation till birth is called a fetus. In the examination of a fetus following questions are to be answered.

1. What is the intrauterine age of the fetus?
2. Whether the fetus was viable or not?
3. Whether there is any sign of survival?
4. What is the cause of death?

AGE OF THE FETUS (FIGS 9.1 TO 9.3)

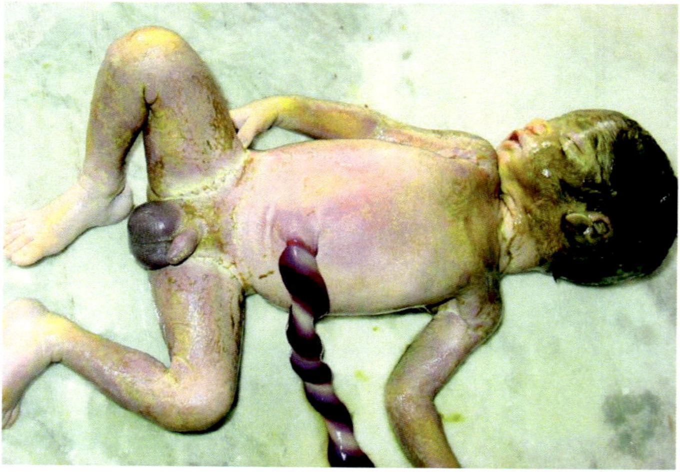

FIGURE 9.1: Age of the fetus can be determined by its length, weight, length of head hair, area of presence or absence of lanugo hair, position of umbilicus, relative development of scrotum with penis, presence of testes, position and development of vulva, labia minora and majora, growth and development of finger and toe nails.

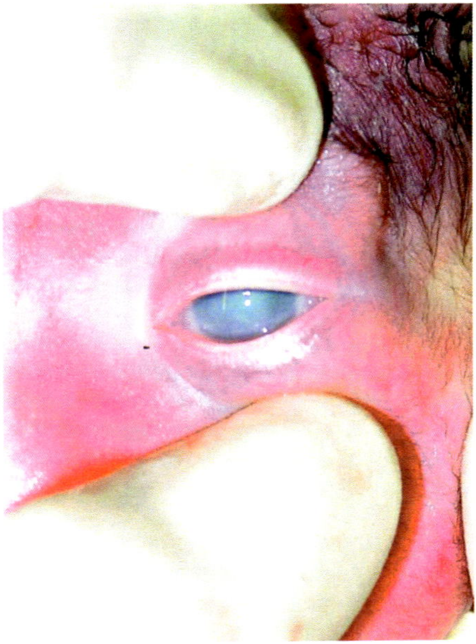

FIGURE 9.2: Examination of eyes of the fetus is important to determine age of viability. Eyes should be examined for separation of eyelids and presence of pupillary membrane.

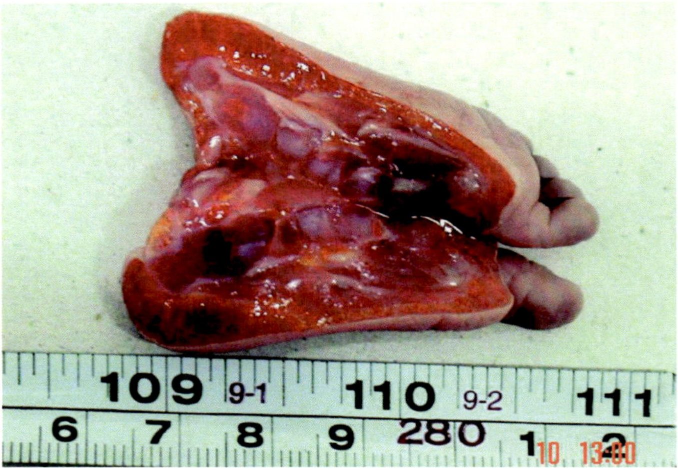

FIGURE 9.3: Examination of centers appearing in the foot and lower end of femur are important for age determination. Center for calcaneum appears at the end of fifth month while that for talus appears at the end of sixth month. Center for lower end of femur appears at ninth month. It is advisable to take a whole body X-ray of the fetus to visualize the appeared centers.

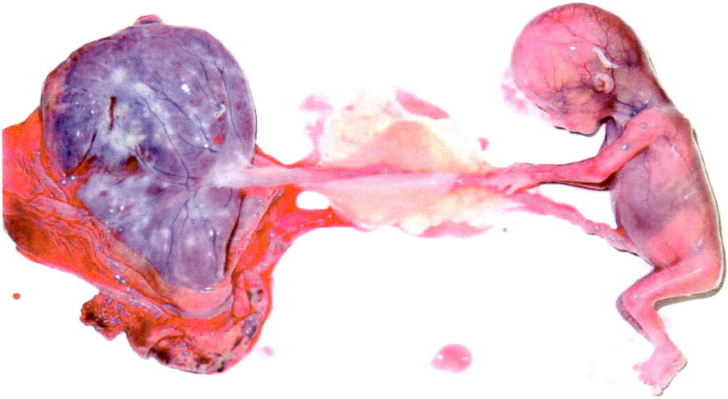

FIGURE 9.4: If the fetus is present with umbilical cord and placenta then length of umbilical cord and, weight and diameter of placenta should be measured. Placenta should be examined for any abnormality.

VIABILITY OF FETUS (FIG. 9.4)

If the estimated age of the fetus is more than 28 weeks then it is a viable fetus.

SIGNS OF SURVIVAL (FIGS 9.5 AND 9.6)

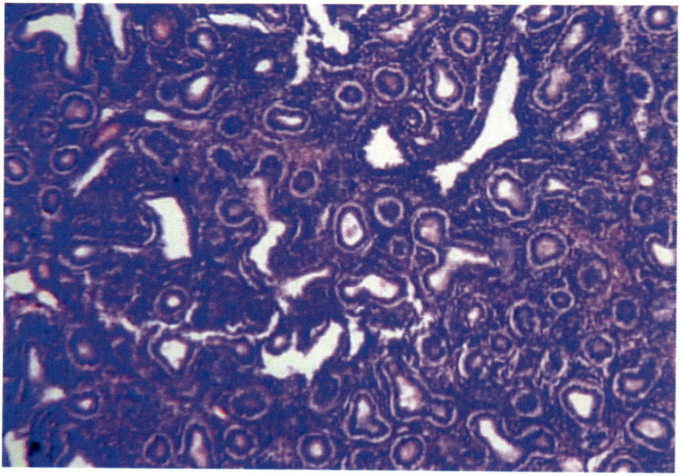

FIGURE 9.5: Signs of respiration indicate that the fetus had survived till birth. This can be established by floating lung and its pieces in water at hydrostatic test and histological study of lung. An un-respired lung is a glandular structure on histology (X100 H and E stain).

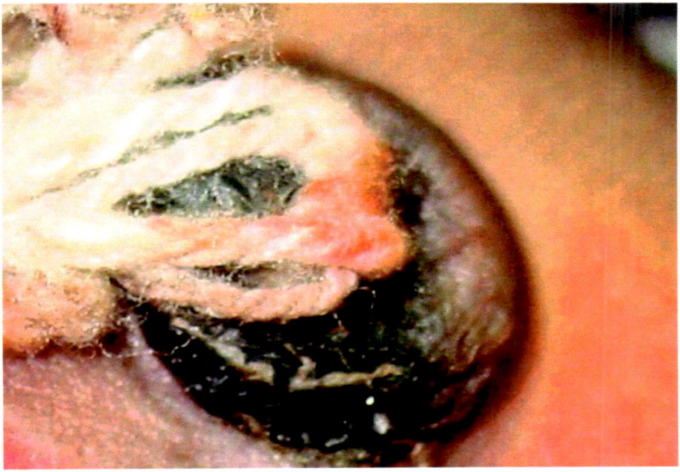

FIGURE 9.6: Dried shriveled stump of umbilical cord with signs of healing at umbilicus is a confirmatory sign of survival.

Similarly presence of curd in stomach is a confirmatory sign of survival.

CAUSE OF DEATH

This question is to be answered when it is established that the fetus was viable and had survived. The common causes of death are head injury, multiple injuries, smothering, etc.

10 Poisoning

It is death caused by local and/or systemic action of poison introduced in the body.

The local action of poison depends on its chemical property. It may be mild to severe irritant or mild to severe corrosive. The systemic action of the poison depend on its components which gets absorbed in the body without change or after certain chemical changes. For instance sulfuric acid gives local reaction depending on its concentration. If it is concentrated (more than 80%) then it gives fumes. So if the acid is consumed, the victim will receive corrosions to gastrointestinal tract as well as to the respiratory tract by the fumes. The absorbed sulfuric acid gets dissociated into H^+ and SO_4^- ions. Both ions have no systemic action. H^+ is normal component of blood and SO_4^- is normally used as a base in many medicines and it has no systemic reaction. However if the consumed sulfuric acid is in dilute form it causes corrosion of gastrointestinal tract and do not cause any damages to respiratory tract unless and until it is aspirated in it.

Poisoning may be suspected in all sudden deaths, negative autopsies and decomposed bodies without any evidence of injury. Examination of clothes should be conducted in respect to any peculiar smell and stains of poisonous material or vomits. Hands should be examined for stains or smell of the poison.

EXTERNAL FINDINGS (FIGS 10.1 AND 10.2)

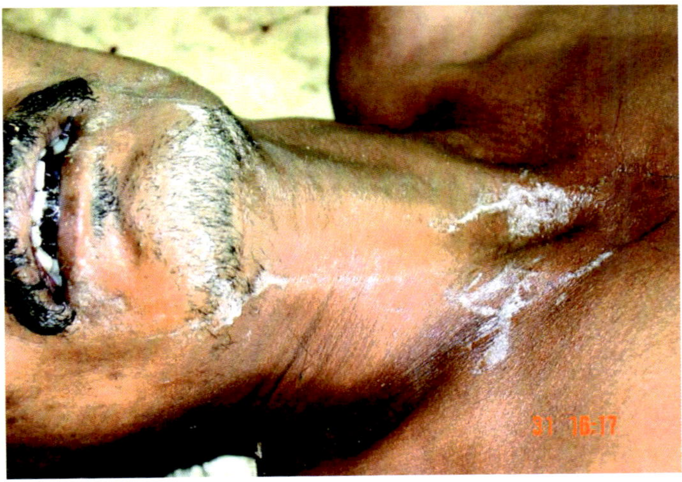

FIGURE 10.1: Examination of face may reveal stain of the poison.

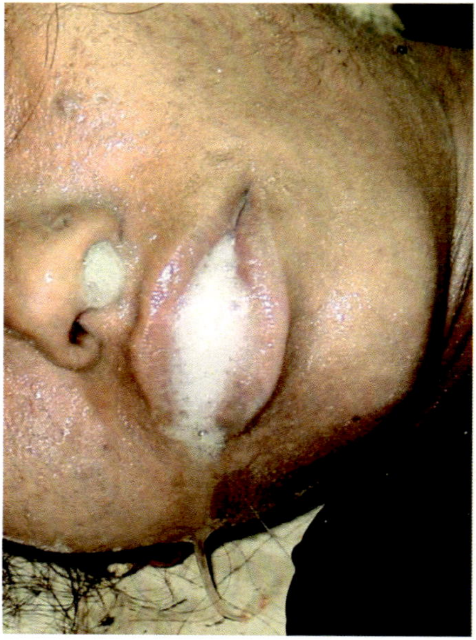

FIGURE 10.2: Froth from mouth and/or nostrils found in the case of poisoning is known to be caused by pulmonary edema.

INTERNAL FINDINGS (FIGS 10.3 TO 10.8)

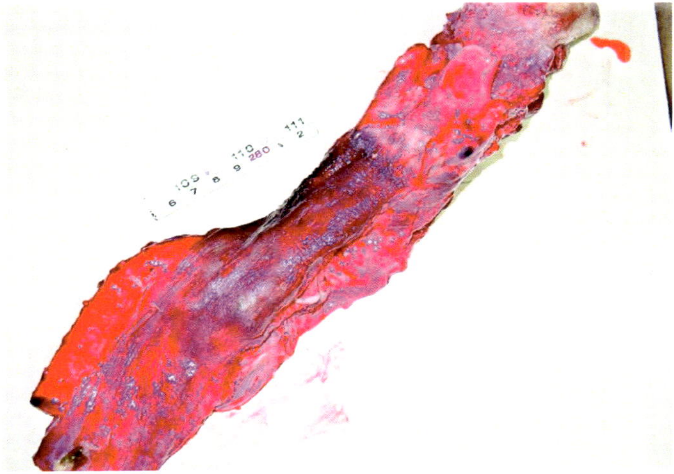

FIGURE 10.3: Damage to esophagus may range from no damage to severe corrosion depending on the chemical property of the poison.

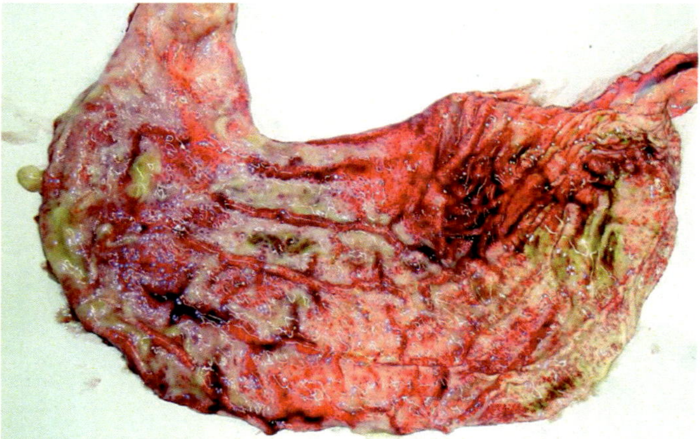

FIGURE 10.4: Damage to stomach mucosa depends on the chemical components of the poison. This picture depicts the erosion of stomach by an organo-phosphorus compound.

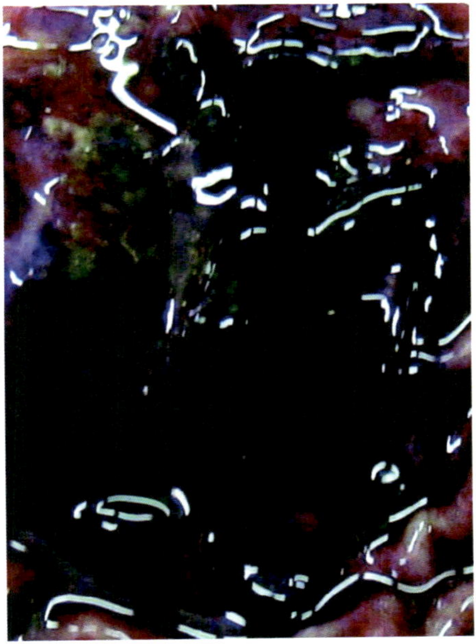

FIGURE 10.5: Carbonization reaction by sulfuric acid.

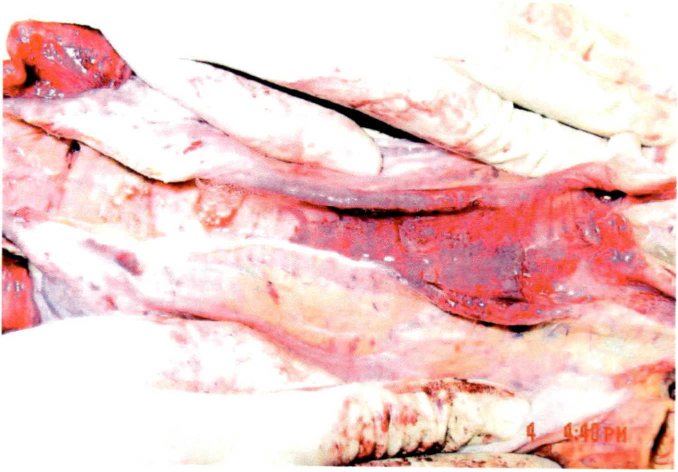

FIGURE 10.6: Inhalation of the fumes of sulfuric acid cause erosion of mucosa of complete respiratory tract. This finding is very rare and depends on the concentration of fumes in air which ultimately depend on the concentration of acid.

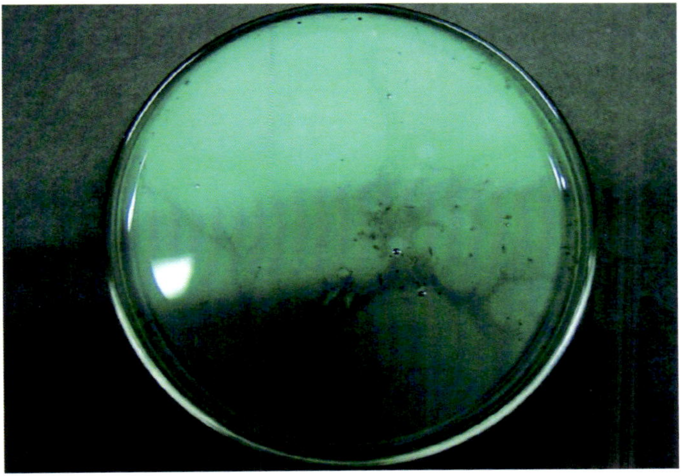

FIGURE 10.7: Contents of the stomach should be examined for their smell (with caution), consistency, color and amount. It should be preserved for toxicological analysis in a suitable preservative.

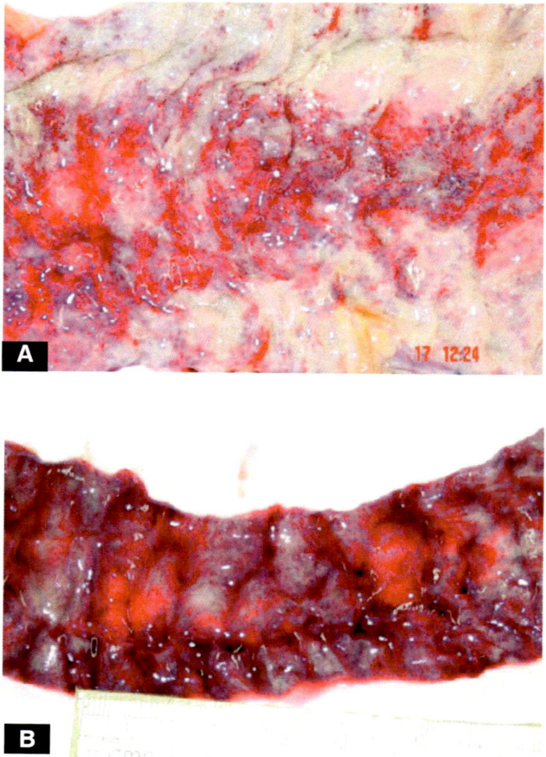

FIGURES 10.8A AND B: Presence of poison in small and/or large intestine confirms that death is most probably caused due to poisoning. However the final opinion must be delivered after toxicological analysis.

OTHER FINDINGS (FIGS 10.9 TO 10.13)

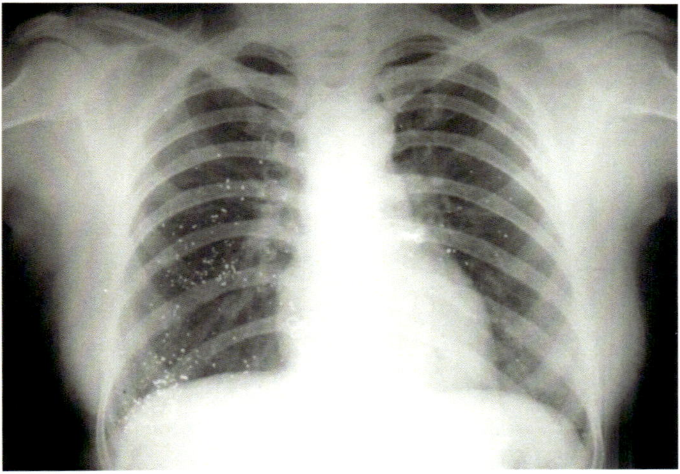

FIGURE 10.9: Radiography is important and diagnostic investigation in heavy metal poisons.

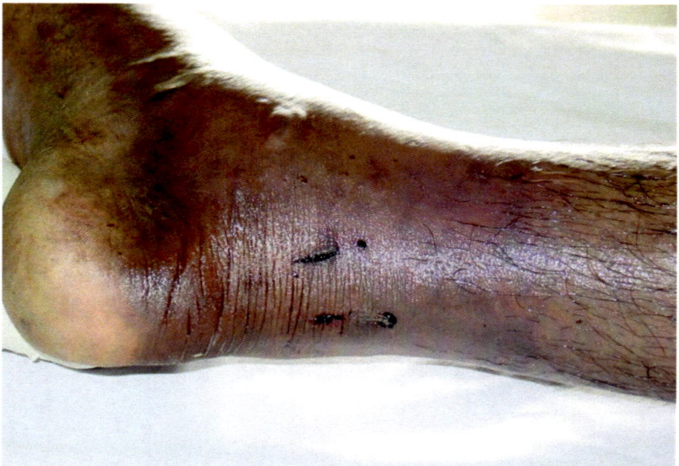

FIGURE 10.10: Fang marks are commonly seen in viper bites. Multiple fang marks must be differentiated from teeth mark of non-poisonous snake. See for the local reaction which indicates severity of envenomation.

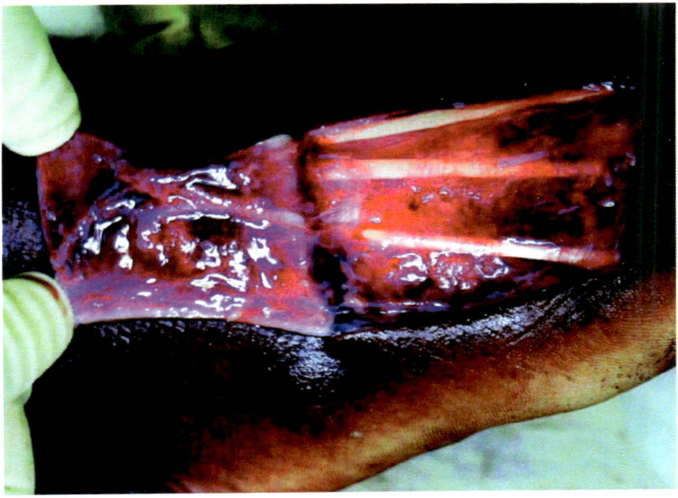

FIGURE 10.11: Sometimes the fang marks cannot be found on external examination. However internal examination reveals the injury to the tissue.

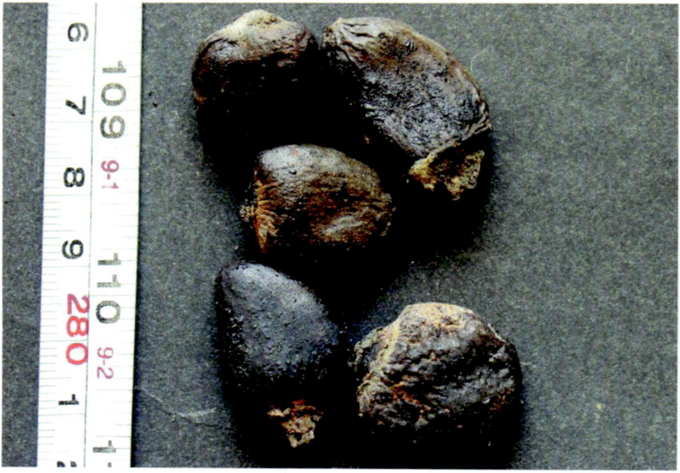

FIGURE 10.12: Marking nut is commonly known for creating injuries by its juice.

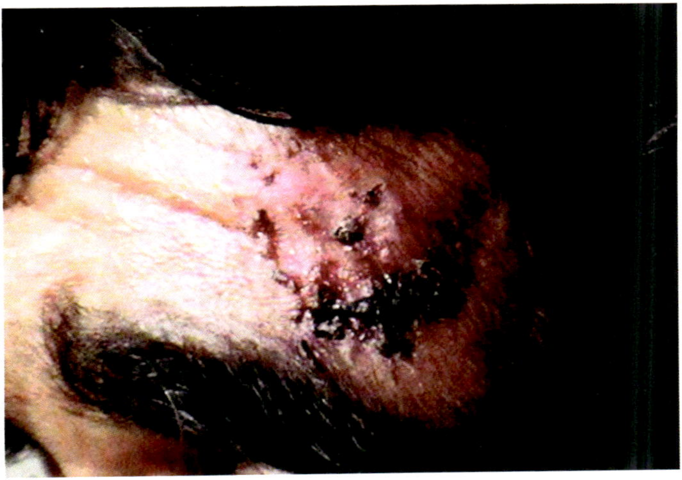

FIGURE 10.13: The injuries caused by irritant marking nut juice seems first like contusion then like abrasion. (*Courtesy:* Dr Kailash U Zine, Associate Professor, Forensic Medicine, Govt. Medical College, Aurangabad).

Smell of alcohol can be detected in CSF, cut sections of organs, contents of stomach and cavities if the person had consumed it before death.

11 Death in Pregnancy

Medicolegal autopsies on pregnant victims are usually carried out when the deceased is brought as a case of sudden death, death followed by delivery or abortion.

The questions which are supposed to be answered are:

1. Is she pregnant?
2. What is the period of pregnancy?
3. What is the cause of death?

EXTERNAL EXAMINATION (FIGS 11.1 TO 11.5)

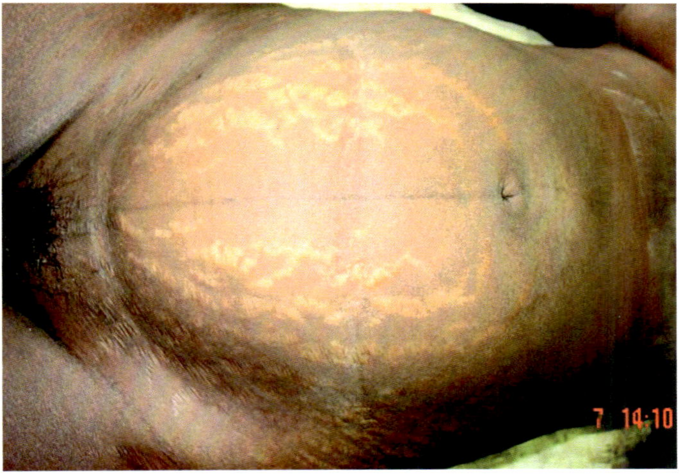

FIGURE 11.1: Many times the external signs of pregnancy are obvious. However they are difficult to notice in a primipara at first trimester. There may not be any history available if the victim is unmarried. Linea alba and linea nigra can be seen in advanced pregnancy.

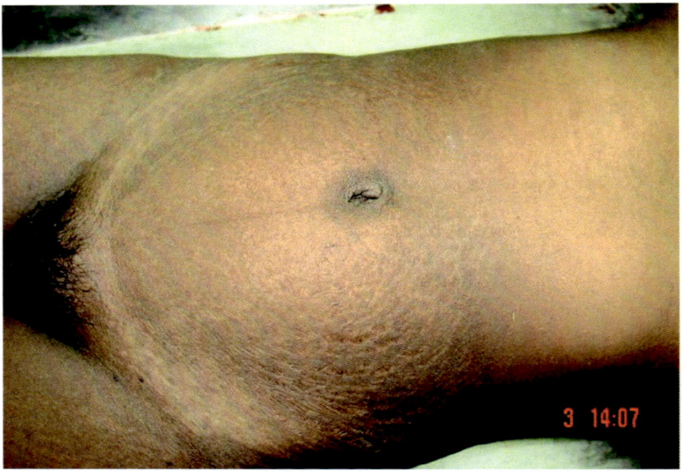

FIGURE 11.2: In recent delivery the abdomen wall is lax, wrinkled and striae gravidarum may be found.

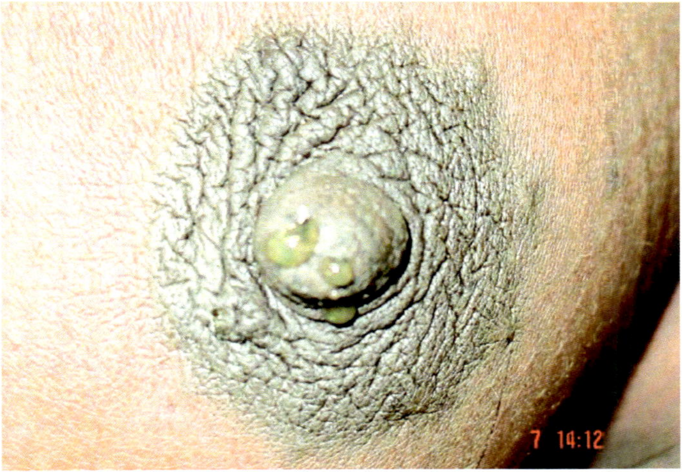

FIGURE 11.3: Examination of breast may reveal enlargement of breast with dark pigmentation of nipple and dark colored tubercles of the enlarged sebaceous glands after second month of pregnancy. Colostrum can be expressed by compression of breast from periphery towards center after third month of pregnancy.

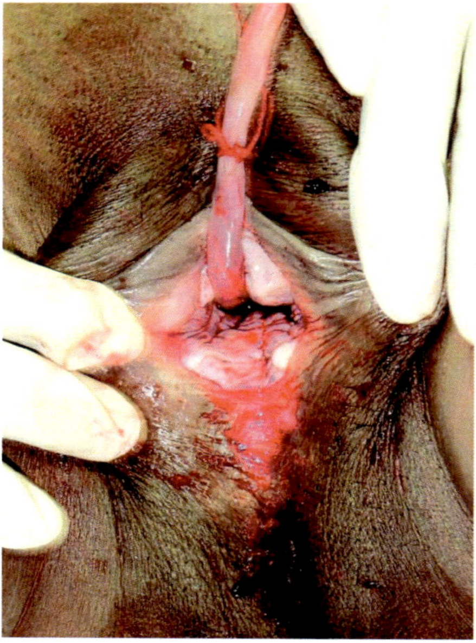

FIGURE 11.4: Genital examination may reveal gross lacerations of perineum and vaginal wall when the delivery is unassisted or assisted by untrained person.

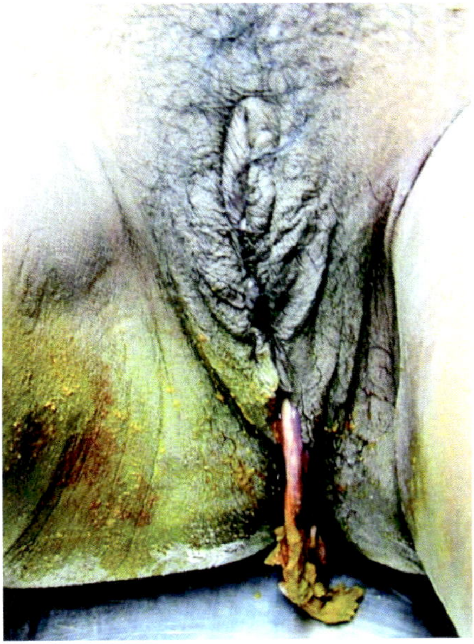

FIGURE 11.5: Turmeric powder or lime or mixture of both may be found applied over injuries and/or severed umbilical cord in deliveries at home or when they are not assisted by medical staff. In this case the torn retained placental membrane is seen protruding out.

INTERNAL EXAMINATION (FIGS 11.6 TO 11.12)

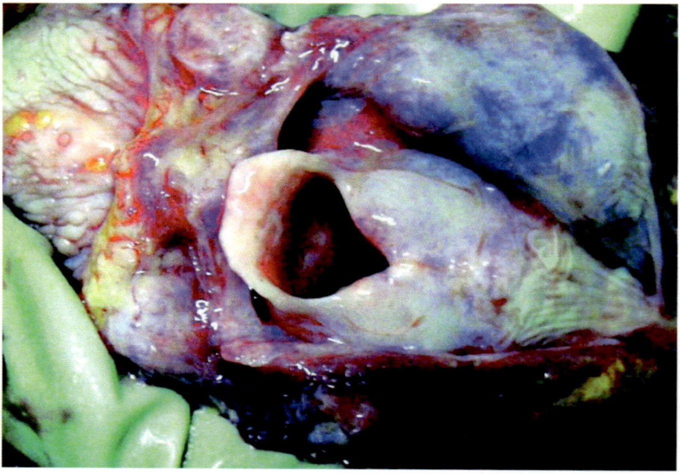

FIGURE 11.6: Internal examination commonly reveals edema of larynx and lung.

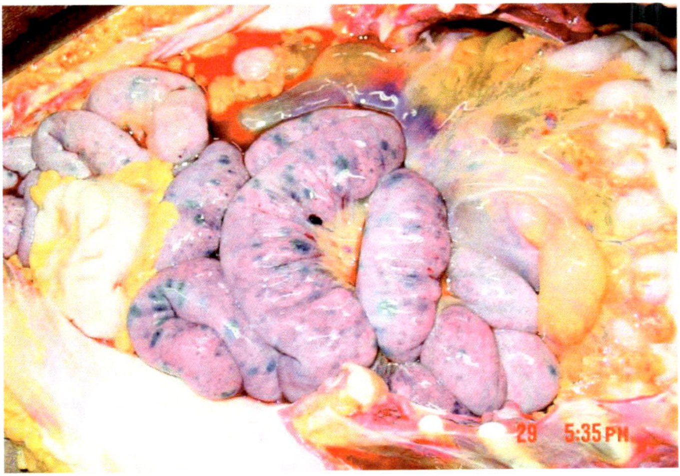

FIGURE 11.7: All organs must be examined for hemorrhages, necrotic areas and edema. Disseminated intravascular coagulopathy (DIC), sickle cell crisis, hemorrhagic shock, amniotic embolism are causes of sudden maternal death. Trauma, toxicological and histological study must be done in all maternal deaths. This photo depicts hemorrhages in intestinal wall in a case of DIC.

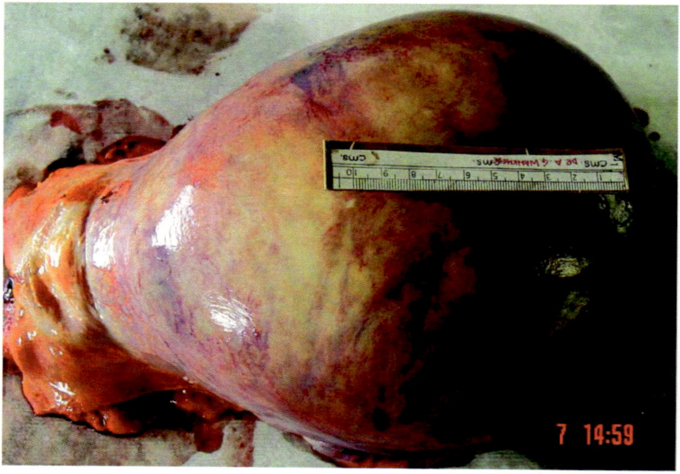

FIGURE 11.8: Uterus should be dissected out with fallopian tubes, ovaries and cervix along with distal half of vaginal wall. All measurements with weight should be taken before dissection.

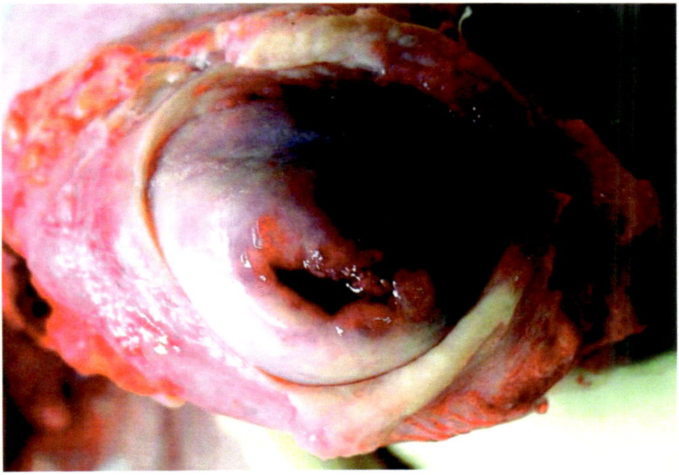

FIGURE 11.9: Vaginal wall and cervix is to be examined along with external surface of uterus for any injury or pathology.

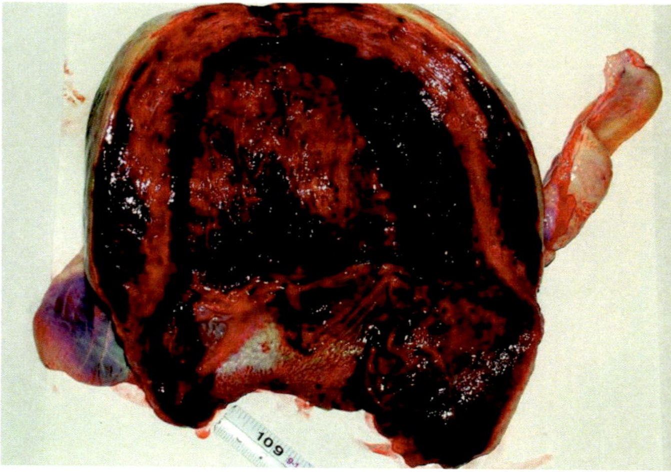

FIGURE 11.10: The uterine cavity may reveal products of conception, clots, and parts of product of conception and/or foreign body. This photograph shows retained placental membrane, one of the common causes of uterine hemorrhage.

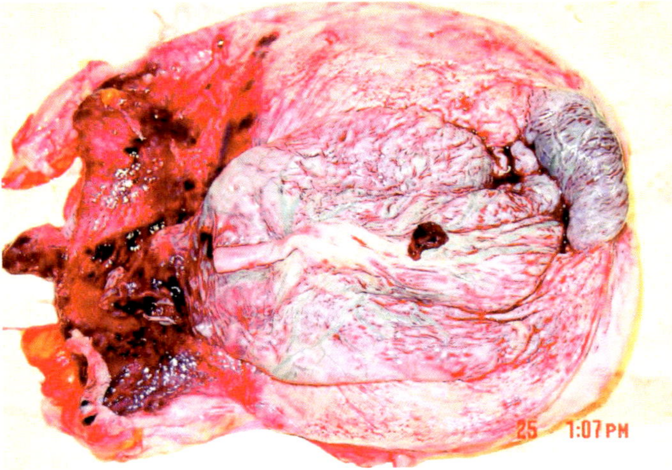

FIGURE 11.11: If the placenta is *in situ* then its site of attachment must be noticed with the condition of membrane.

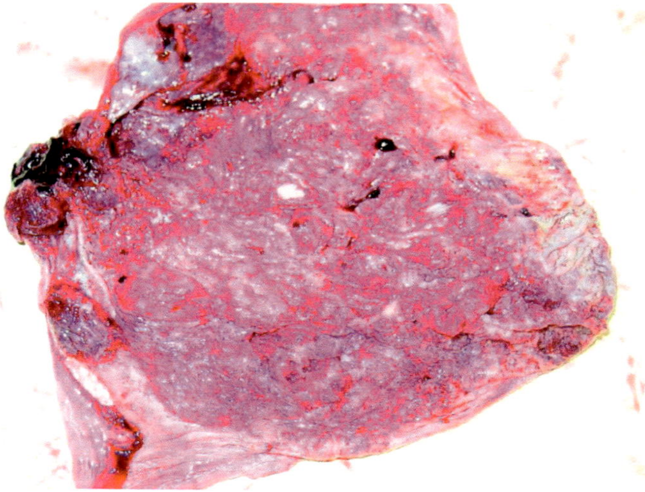

FIGURE 11.12: The placenta should be examined after removal from uterus. The inner lining of uterus and placenta should be examined grossly and histologically.

12 Sudden Death

Sudden death is death due to unexpected and undiagnosed disease or condition. They are either pathological or physiological conditions. However, after conducting autopsy, before concluding the opinion as a natural death, chemical and toxicological analysis is advisable. Some other special investigations, circumstantial evidences and history of past illness should be considered before opining about the cause of death. Many cases of sudden death are either due to the system or multi-system involvement. Cardiovascular, nervous or respiratory system diseases are common causes of sudden deaths.

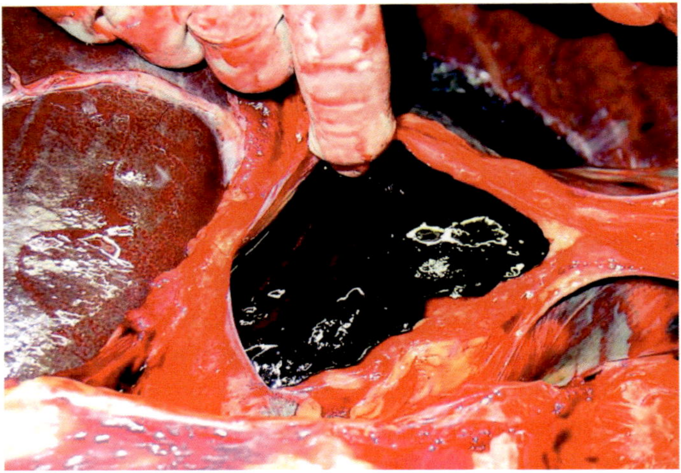

FIGURE 12.1: Cardiac tamponade due to rupture of old myocardial infarction or rupture of aneurysm of ascending part of aorta is one of the causes of sudden death. Rupture of aortic aneurysm at any part can cause sudden death.

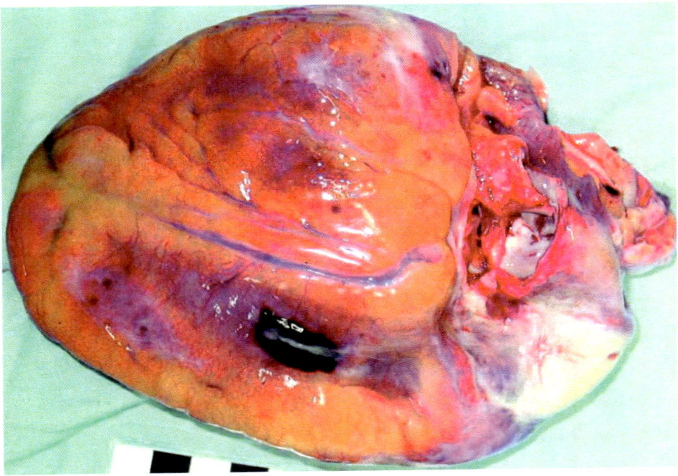

FIGURE 12.2: Myocardial infarction is the commonest cause of sudden death. This photograph shows a twenty-eight hours old myocardial infarct. However this type of finding is seldom seen in these cases as the victims succumb before any grossly detectable changes in heart.

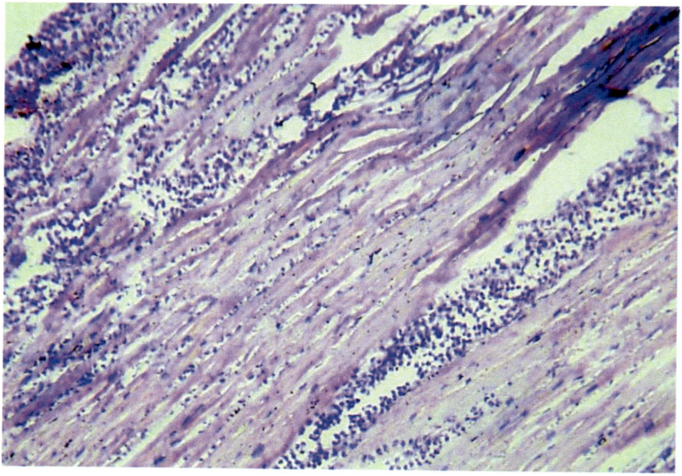

FIGURE 12.3: Microscopically a myocardial infarction show eosinophilia, cardiac muscle swelling, cell membrane blurring, cytoplasmic granularity, waviness of cardiac muscle and increased interstitial cells after about six hours of survival following myocardial infarct (X100 H and E stain).

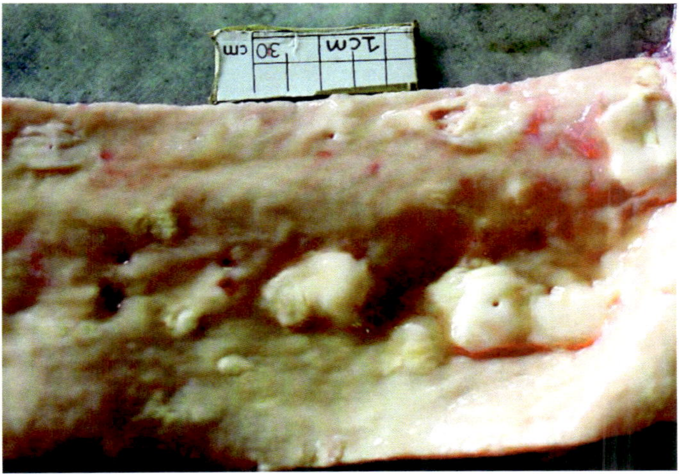

FIGURE 12.4: Large arteries and coronaries should be examined for blockage and atherosclerotic changes.

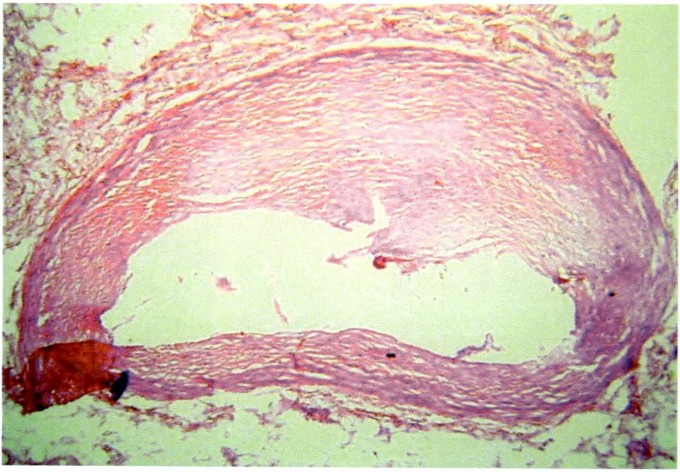

FIGURE 12.5: Microscopic examination of atherosclerotic plaque in a coronary is necessary to detect recent hemorrhages. Here there is no hemorrhage.

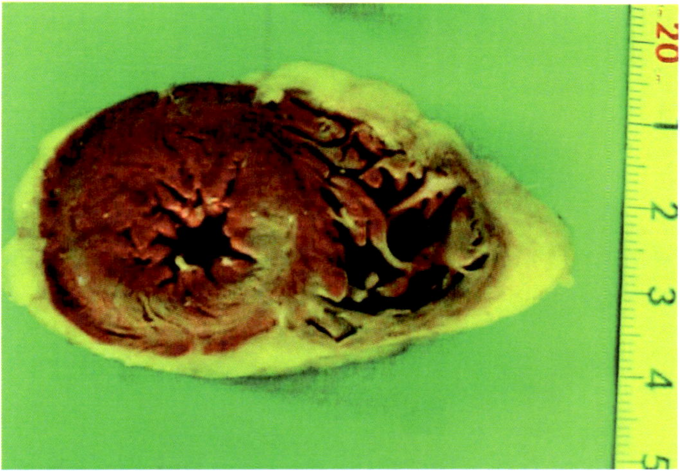

FIGURE 12.6: Gross histochemical staining technique such as TTC (Triphenyltetrazolium chloride) and/or fluorescent microscopy is helpful to detect areas of myocardial infarcts of less than six hours. However, its fallacies should be considered along with all other investigations before finalizing opinion about cause of death.

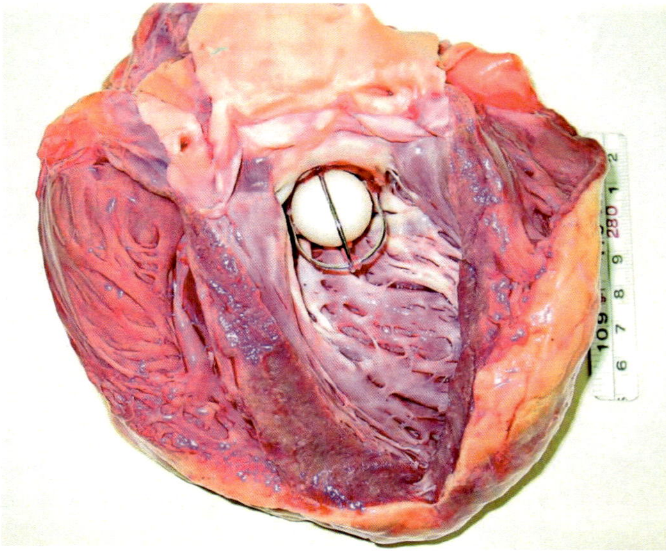

FIGURE 12.7: Previous surgical management of heart should be notified.

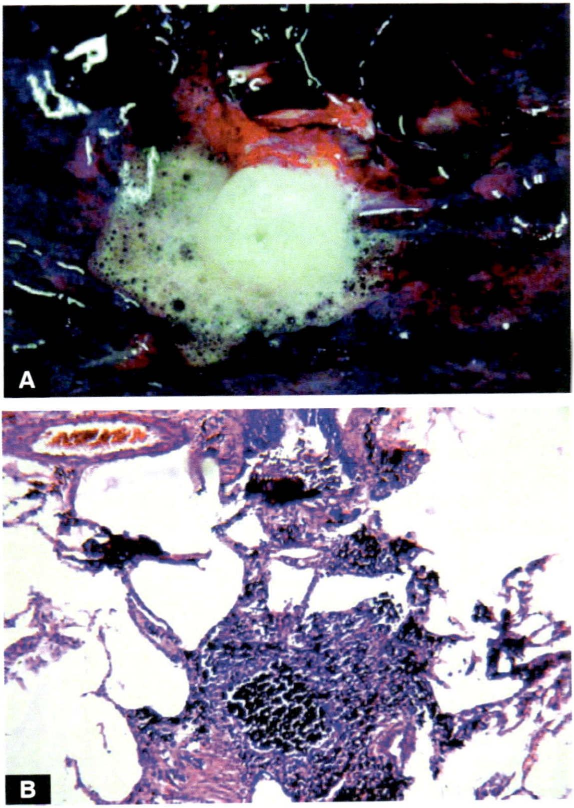

FIGURES 12.8A AND B: Pulmonary edema is one of the fastest killers. However one must try to find out its cause.

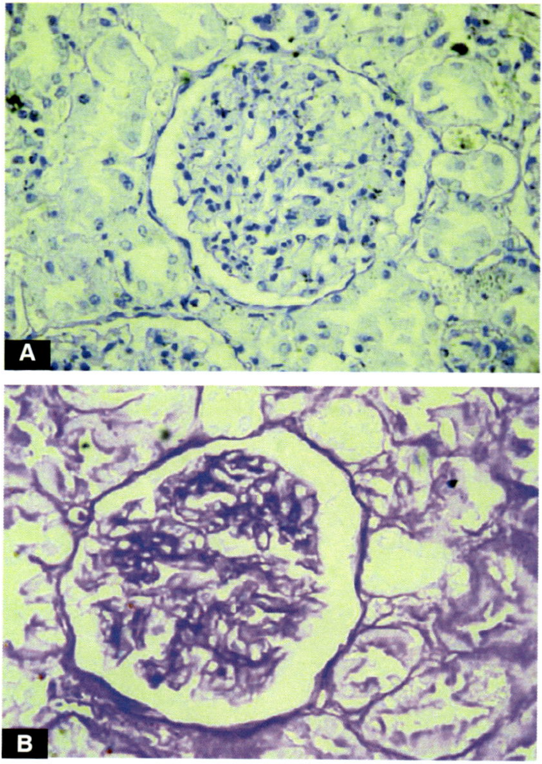

FIGURES 12.9A AND B: In all deaths associated with diabetes, histological study of kidney is necessary to determine thickness of basement membrane with other changes. In this case the basement membrane is normal (X400 PAS staining).

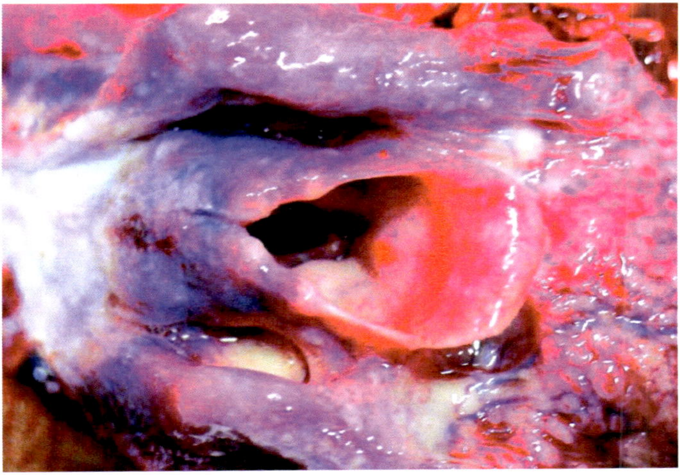

FIGURE 12.10: Laryngeal edema is known to cause sudden death. Drugs, allergens, anaphylaxis, etc. are known causes.

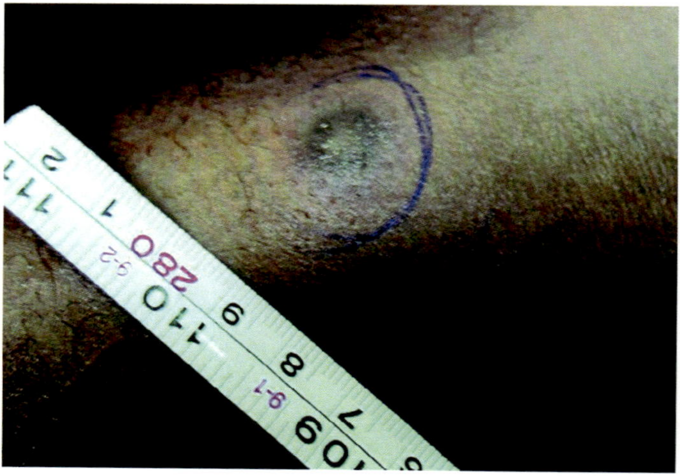

FIGURE 12.11: Anaphylactic reaction is known to cause sudden death. If the anaphylaxis is caused during medical treatment by a known drug causing anaphylaxis it is very important to note whether sensitivity test was done or not. Its absence or presence will determine whether the treating doctor was negligent or not. The site of injection mark from where the drug was administered should be preserved for histopathology study and chemical analysis with control skin.

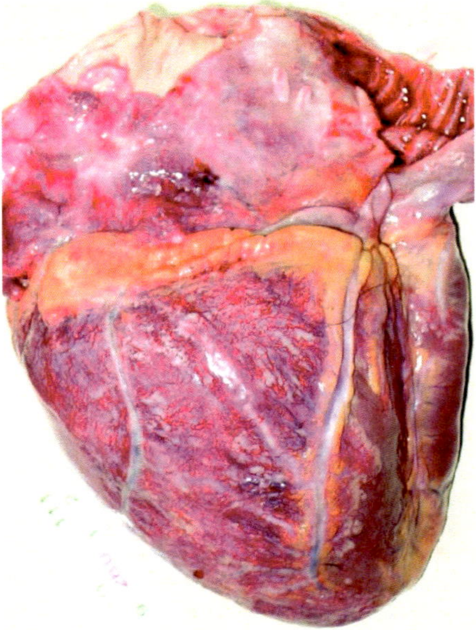

FIGURE 12.12: Evidence of the disease for which the drug was administered is to be searched for. This photograph shows pericarditis as a disease for which the drug was administered. Histological study of all organs including adrenal glands should be done.

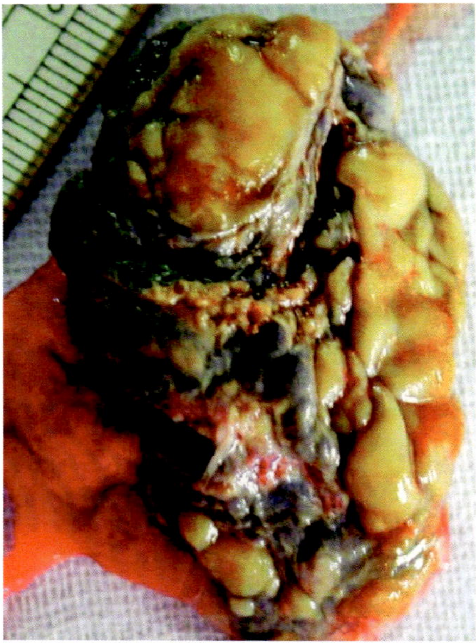

FIGURE 12.13: Sickle cell crisis is a known cause of sudden death. Findings like autosplenectomy or multiple scars in the parenchyma of spleen can be found in these cases. However the diagnosis of death by sickle cell crisis depends on microinfarcts in the organs including skin with presence of sickled RBCs and not merely on the presence of sickled RBCs on histological study.

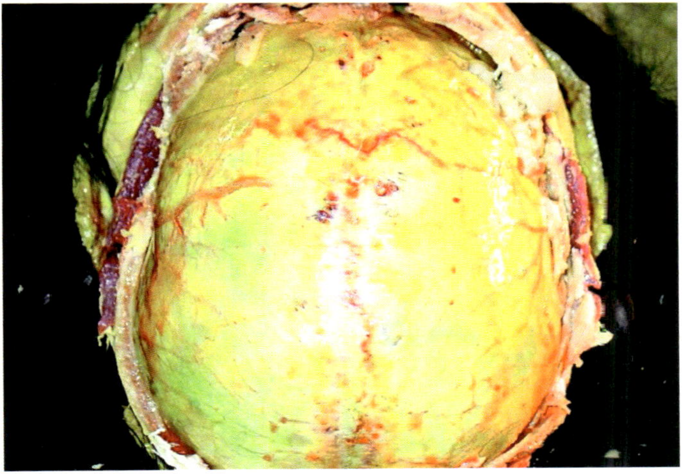

FIGURE 12.14: Hepatitis is also known to cause sudden death. In extreme cases almost all protein rich contents of the body are yellow in color. Here the dura mater is shown.

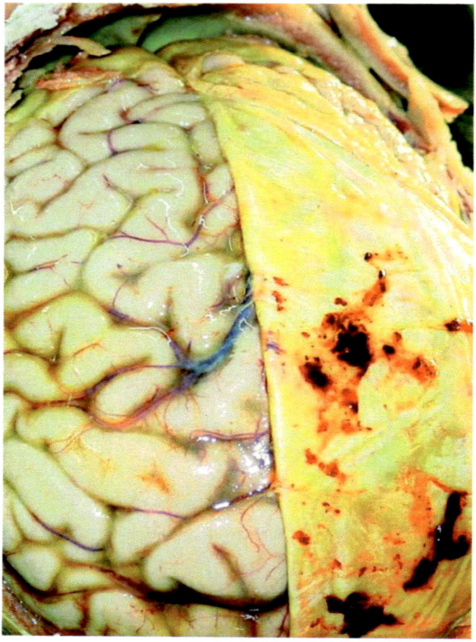

FIGURE 12.15: The inner surface of dura revealed multiple areas of hemorrhages in the case shown in Figure 12.14. Note the yellow color of CSF.

13 Injuries in Sexual Violence

The usual target area in sexual violence is breast and vagina. However complete body examination is essential. Neck, lips, mouth and anus can be the targeted areas of violence. Evidences and samples should be collected from all these sites.

Examination of clothes for damage, stains and foreign bodies is vital part in deaths associated with sexual violence. They should be air dried and, packed in paper bag followed by plastic bag with small holes to avoid decomposition and destruction of biological material on the clothes. Pubic hair should be examined for matting and combed for foreign hair. They should be collected by cutting with scissors. Swabs should be collected from perineum, vagina, cervix, anus, mouth and nipples. A smear on clean glass slide should be prepared from each swab. One should try to avoid contamination of site examined and sample by gloves. All swabs and smears should be air dried and then each swab should be kept in a dry test tube or bottle and corked. All slides should be examined under microscope for intact sperm or head of sperm. They should be kept in a box after indicating their site of collection.

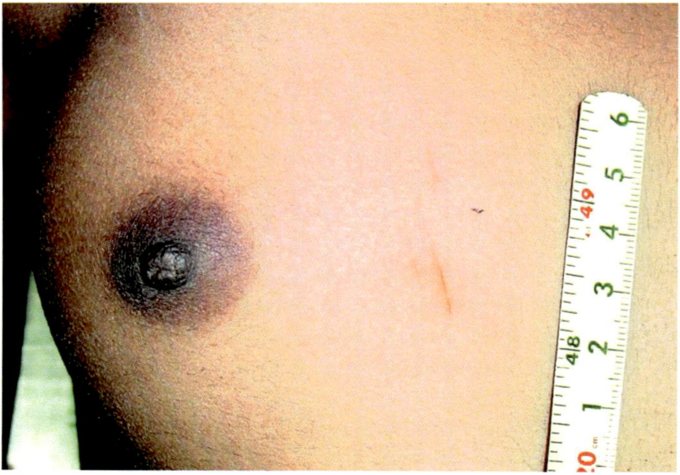

FIGURE 13.1: Examination of breast may reveal scratch abrasions over breast.

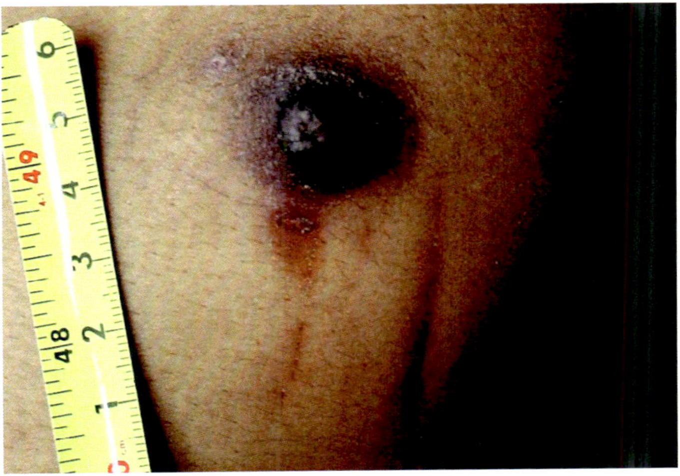

FIGURE 13.2: Nipples may be bitten or squeezed. The skin of nipple may be abraded. A swab must be collected from this type of injuries for further investigation. Note the difference between the nipples in previous figure with this.

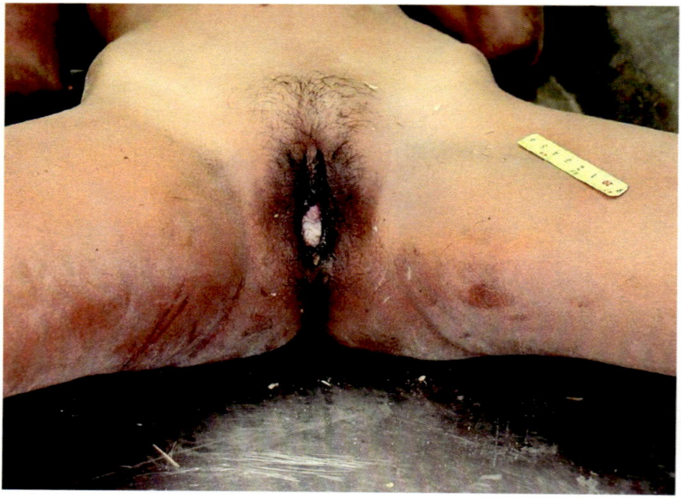

FIGURE 13.3: Examination of external genitalia is of much importance. In non-consensual sexual intercourse there is always some damage to the genitalia. What is required is a very meticulous examination. Bruises and abrasions can be seen on the medial aspect of thighs. Vulva may show bruises. Vaginal and perineal lacerations should be noticed properly in respect to position of examination and clock wise position.

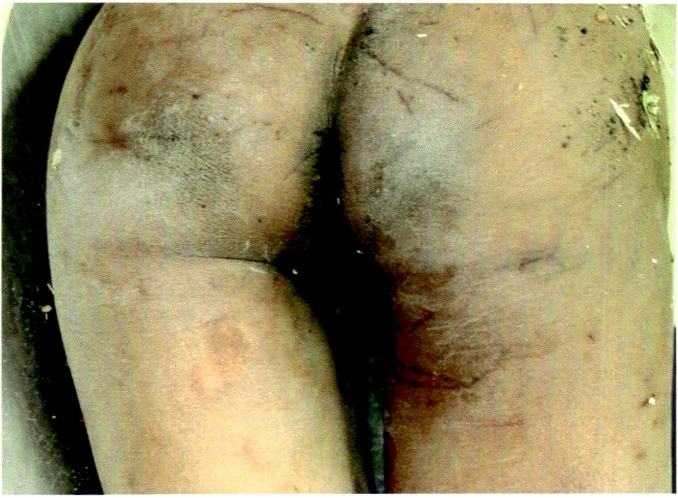

FIGURE 13.4: Examination of buttocks and back also is very important as it reveals the underlying area and surface on which the victim was lying in the act of sexual intercourse. It also shows signs of violence in the form of injuries. Blood and semen can be found collected in the gluteal fold or around anus if the victim was lying on back after sexual intercourse and death.

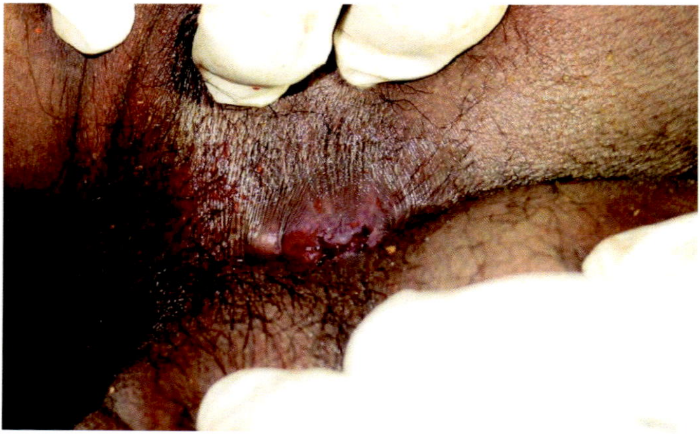

FIGURE 13.5: This photograph reveals postmortem bleeding from hemorrhoids in a case of hanging which was considered as a case of anal sexual violence followed by suicide. There was no sign of any damage, lubrication, chronic anal intercourse or impalement to anus or peri-anal area.

14 Artifacts

These are the damages caused to the victim or deceased which may be misunderstood and misinterpreted. Understanding artifacts is of very much importance to avoid disastrous problems.

ARTIFACTS DUE TO RESUSCITATION (FIGS 14.1 TO 14.3)

Increase in the numbers of hospitals and use of machines in medical science brought in different types of injuries.

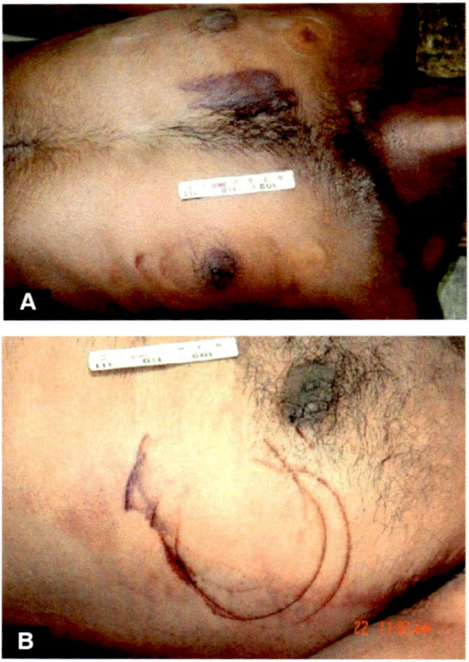

FIGURES 14.1A AND B: Intra-cardiac injection marks, fractures of ribs in anterior chest wall and damages around mouth and nose during artificial breathing may be mistaken for antemortem injury. Nowadays abrasions caused by defibrillators are the commonest one. The shape and distribution of these injuries are very peculiar. The underlying tissue show very minimal or no damages as compared to those caused with same force before dying.

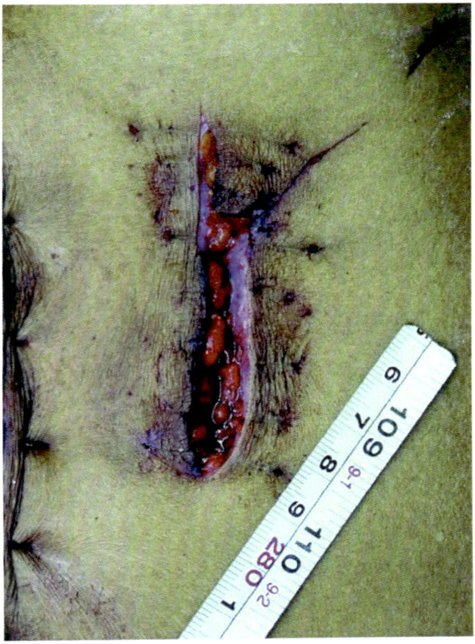

FIGURE 14.2: Surgical injuries may be considered as injuries of violence. The stab injury with tailing in this figure is darker in color than the surgical wound which is lighter in color.

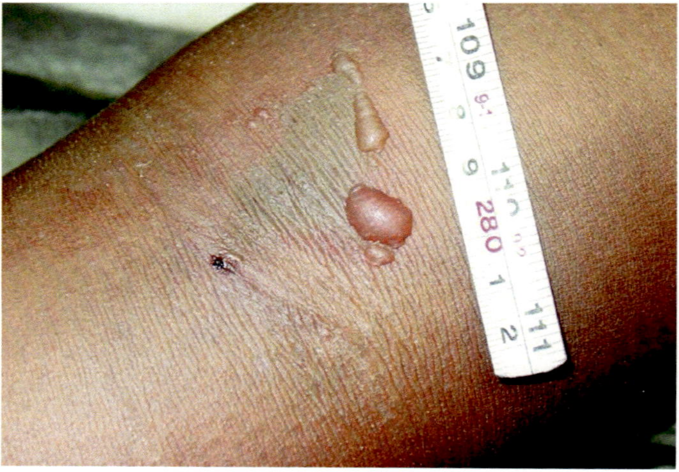

FIGURE 14.3: Vesicle and extravasation of blood at the site of injection can be seen in many cases. It should not be mistaken for burn or bruise.

ARTIFACTS DUE TO POSTMORTEM CHANGES (FIGS 14.4 TO 14.10)

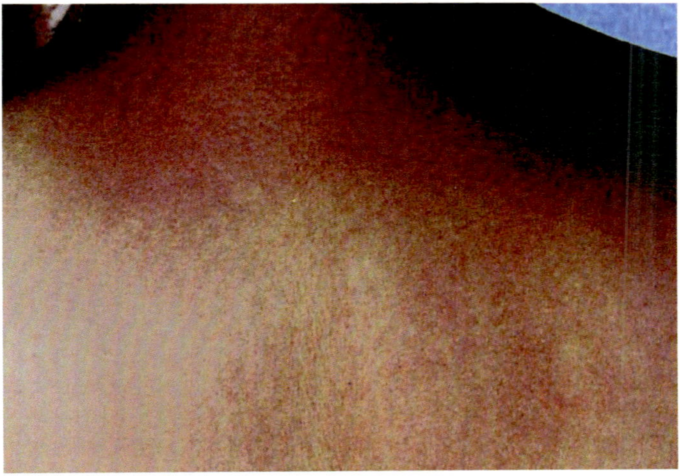

FIGURE 14.4: Certain injuries like first degree burns giving rise to mere redness when alive or bruises causing mere hyperemia in the area where the blunt force is applied may be noted by the inquest conducting officer in his report. With passing time these injuries cannot be seen by postmortem conducting medical practitioner as they are in the region of postmortem lividity or the blood from hyperemia shifts to the dependent part of the body. Possibility of such injuries should not be denied at autopsy.

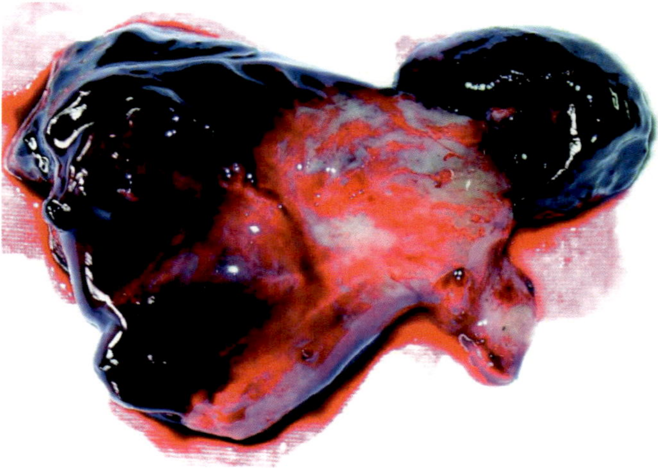

FIGURE 14.5: Postmortem intravascular clotting is a unique phenomenon called as chicken fat clot. The clot has separate cellular and plasma part and they are easily removable from the vessels and heart.

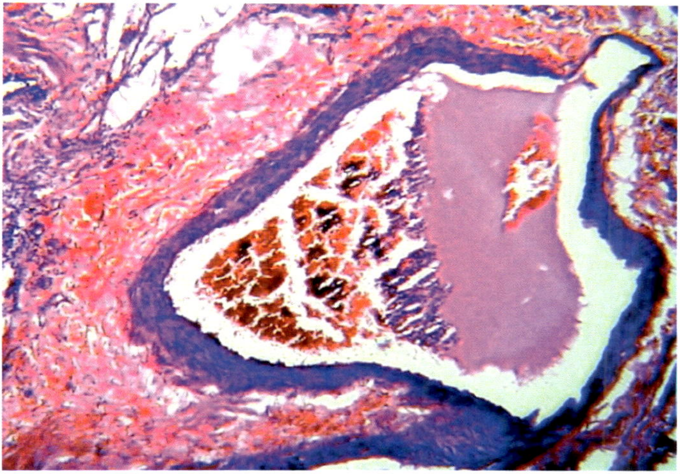

FIGURE 14.6: Features of postmortem clot are easily detectable in the small vessels too. Separated cellular and plasma part can be seen.

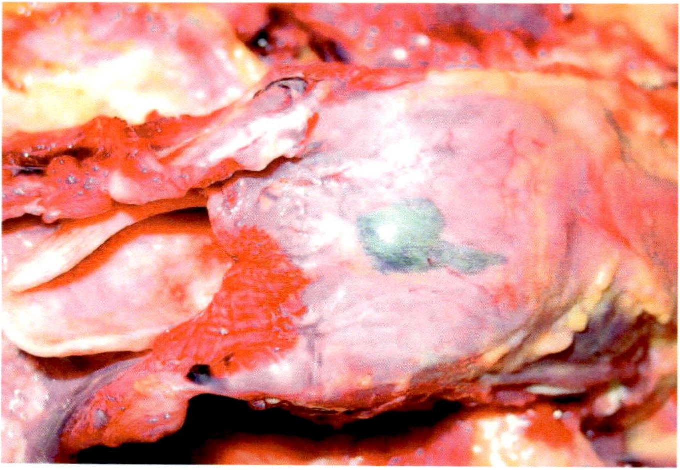

FIGURE 14.7: Collection of blood on the posterior part of esophagus is almost always postmortem in nature. Histological study of the lesion should be carried out if there is any dispute.

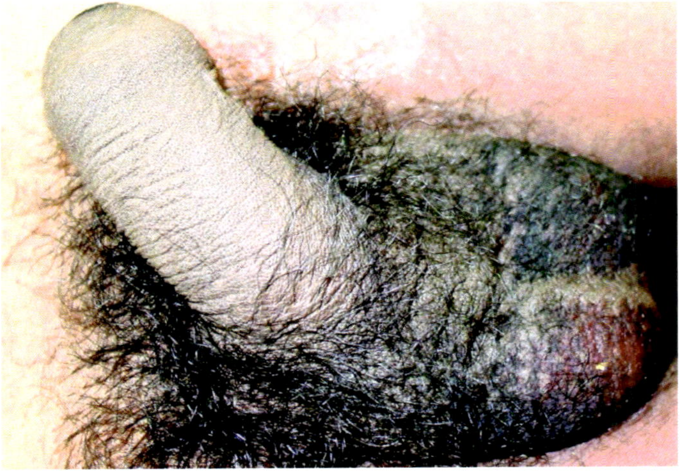

FIGURE 14.8: Scrotal skin is moist in life. The exposed part of it becomes dry following death and may be mistaken as abrasion.

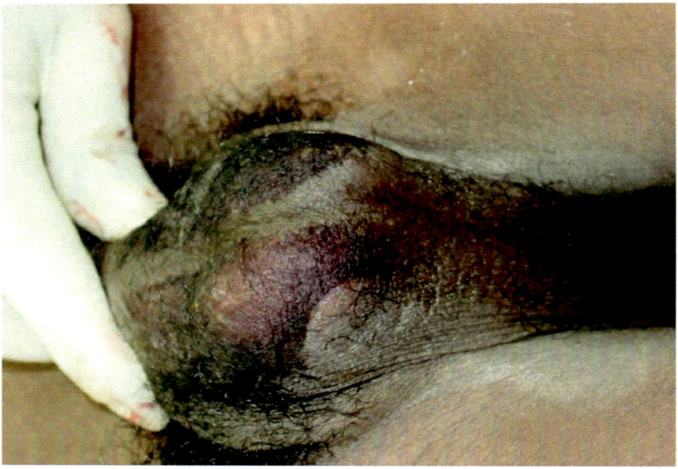

FIGURE 14.9: However the moisture of scrotal skin is retained where it was in touch of thigh and/or perineum and did not show any drying of skin. The internal examination of scrotum did not reveal any injury.

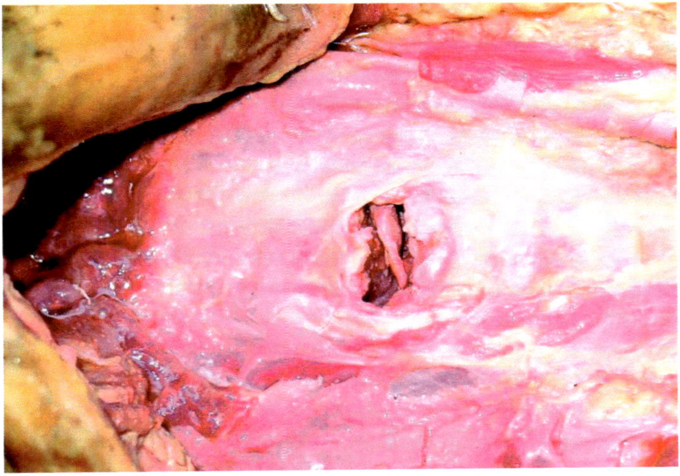

FIGURE 14.10: Decomposition results in shrinkage of cartilages and weakening in articulation. Rough handling of that body part may result in separation of that joint which on dissection looks like fractures. This phenomenon can be seen in spine, laryngeal cartilages, hyoid bone and developing bones.

ARTIFACTS DUE TO INJURIES BY INSECTS AND ANIMALS (FIGS 14.11 TO 14.13)

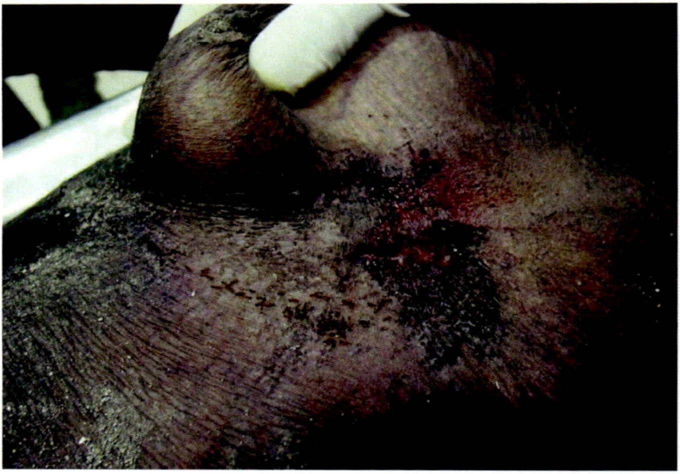

FIGURE 14.11: Ants attack un-decomposed, unprotected dead bodies or unprotected bedridden unconscious patient with un-exfoliated skin. Ants usually attack moist skin at axilla, genitalia, lips, eyelids and margins of folded skin, e.g. lower part of female breast, abdominal and neck folds, etc. While eating superficial skin layers ants secrete their saliva containing formic acid. After some time the ant eaten skin becomes brown due to reaction with formic acid and looks like an abrasion. Presence of live or dead ants on the body usually solves this problem.

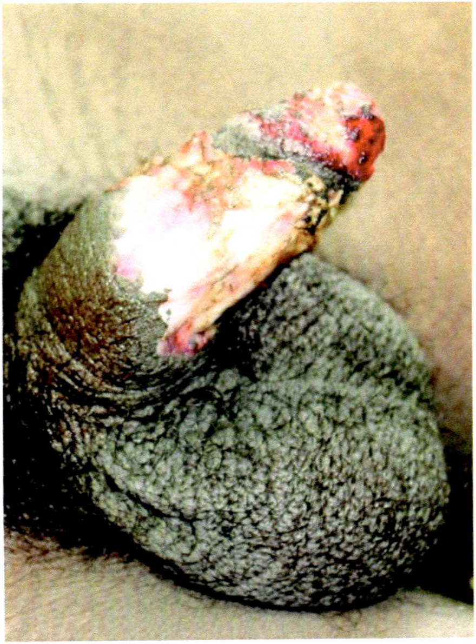

FIGURE 14.12: Rodents are interested in eating soft parts of non-decomposed dead body, e.g. genitalia, lips, eyelids, ears, nose, nipple, etc.

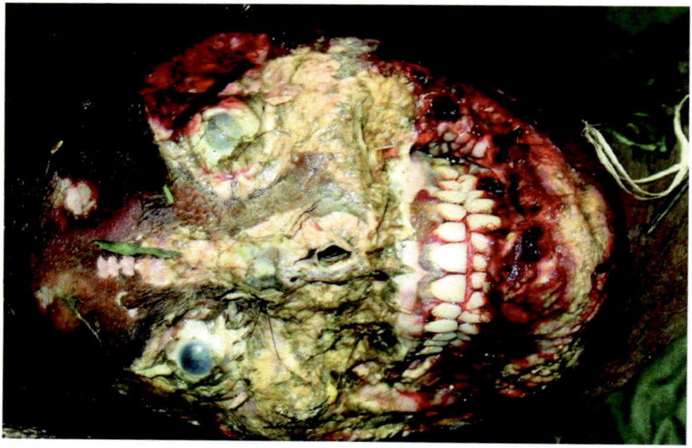

FIGURE 14.13: Aquatic animals usually attack those parts of body which are not covered by clothes and are present under water. Body surface which is in touch with ground under water or floating above water is usually spared.

Part II
Clinical Forensic Medicine

15 Introduction to Clinical Forensic Medicine

CLINICAL FORENSIC MEDICINE

This branch deals with clinical examination of the victims and/or accused. Usually a clinician is involved in these examinations. The history, consent, treatment, investigation and preservation of samples play a most critical role in this medicolegal investigation. Examination of the injured including injuries by physical abuse involving victims like women and children are very important and require knowledge and experience of forensic medicine.

There are many disciplines in law where the age is very significant while implementing any section or act or rule, e.g. consent, contract, rape, marriage, judicial punishment, human trafficking, etc.

Examination of accused and victim of sexual offence is a very important piece of information for the respective cases.

Examination of intoxicated persons is again very important in cases of vehicular accidents and cases of abuse.

Examination of physically abused victim or deceased is usually followed by examination of suspected weapons seized by investigating officer. Although examination of weapon is a part of criminalistics, however the doctor who has examined the victim or deceased is supposed to examine the weapon of offence and opine about whether the injuries are possible due to the weapon examined.

For medicolegal examination first important thing is the requisition letter from the investigating officer for the examination of the said person. Sometimes the treatment records or certificates can be asked by investigating authority after hospitalization or discharge from the hospital. In such cases it is to be informed to the patient or his parents in case he is a minor or whenever the patient is admitted to the hospital, he must be made aware that the treatment record or certificates demanded by investigating authority will be issued for legal purpose.

CONSENT

Before proceeding for the physical examination for medico-legal purpose it is very much essential to take informed written consent. The consent should be in the language of the patient. It should be in a question and answer format. The question should be descriptive regarding methodology and consequences of issuing the said report to police. The answer is to be written below the question and then it should be signed by the patient with date below the signature. The consent should be taken from only that patient who is legally eligible to give consent. Otherwise the consent should be taken from the parents. If the patient is not giving consent, in such situation this fact should be informed to the investigating authority in written. Examination of an alcoholic can be conducted by applying substantial force even if the patient has not given consent.

IDENTIFICATION MARKS

Permanent, unique and presence on the exposed part of body makes a mark an ideal identification mark. Minimum two such identification marks must be mentioned on each medicolegal certificate as there is very remote possibility of having similar marks on other persons. From these marks the person can be identified in the court of law.

HISTORY

It is very essential in clinical forensic medicine to take present and past history about the condition or injuries of the patient.

Other important points include mentioning date and time of examination, writing report in good handwriting, putting signature, designation and complete address of the hospital where the patient is examined.

It should always be remembered that while examining a female in medicolegal cases a female medical attendant (it could be a female nurse, intern or doctor) should be present. The female medical attendant must be acquainted with the procedure of medicolegal examination. If the patient is a minor, then his/her male/female relative if available should be present while examination OR if the female patient request for presence of her female relative which could make her comfortable while examination then in both cases the procedure of examination must be explained to the relative before the examination. The relative's name should be mentioned in the report and he/she should be informed about the same.

Never remove clothes of the patient. Let the patient remove their clothes. If the patient is a minor then let the present relative or parent remove the minor's clothes. If the patient is unconscious in that case the clothes should be removed by cutting them near the stitch lines. The clothes should be preserved for further examination if necessary and hospital clothes should be provided immediately to the patient.

16 Determination of Age

Certifying age of the person is necessary when it is at dispute. In Indian laws and Acts, age in years 7, 12, 15, 16, 18, 21, etc. has importance in some or other context.

Medical examination for determining age consist of three parts:

1. Clinical examination
2. Odontological examination
3. Radiological examination.

CLINICAL EXAMINATION

This examination determines physical development and secondary sexual character development. Height, weight, chest girth at the level of nipple and abdominal girth at the level of navel should be taken into consideration to determine physical development. Pubic hair, axillary hair, facial hair, scalp hair, breast development, development of genitalia, voice, Adam's apple, history of menarche, regularity of the menses, skin, eye, etc. should be considered to determine secondary sexual character.

Puberty starts and ends at ~11 years and ~16 years respectively in girls and, ~13 years and ~18 years respectively in boys. However it must be remembered that pubertal changes depends on socioeconomic, nutritional and mental status of the child, i.e. if all or one of these status are poor then the pubertal changes may be delayed by a year or more and vise versa. Hence it is recommended that the history related to pubertal changes and findings regarding pubertal changes with the status of child must be considered to evaluate the age.

Tanner stages of development are useful to determine age from pubertal changes by considering the available data on beginning of puberty in girls and boys in that region and their socioeconomic, nutritional and mental status.

It must be remembered that pubertal changes is a process and not an event. The amount of time needed to progress from stage II to stage V is between two and three years.

DEVELOPMENT OF SECONDARY SEXUAL CHARACTERISTICS IN GIRLS

Tanner Stages of Breast Development (Figs 16.1 to 16.5)

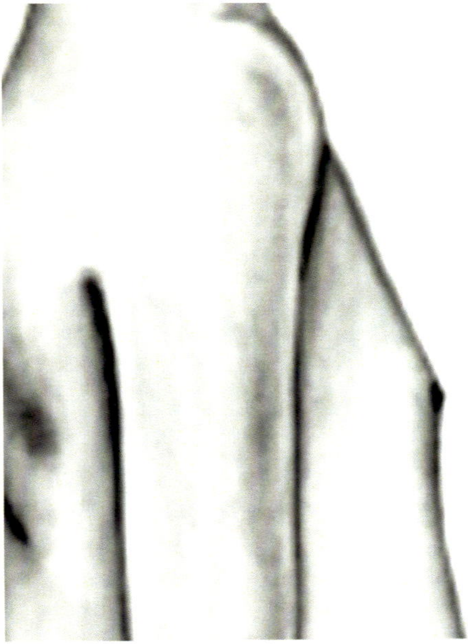

FIGURE 16.1: Stage I, preadolescent, the nipple elevated.

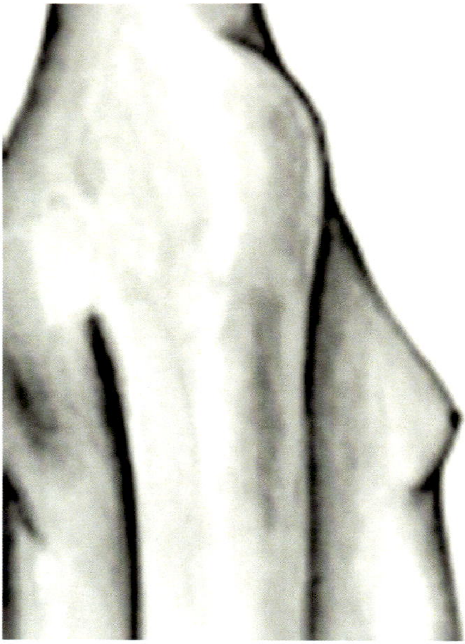

FIGURE 16.2: Stage II, the breast bud develops. The breast tissue and nipple arise as a single mound of tissue.

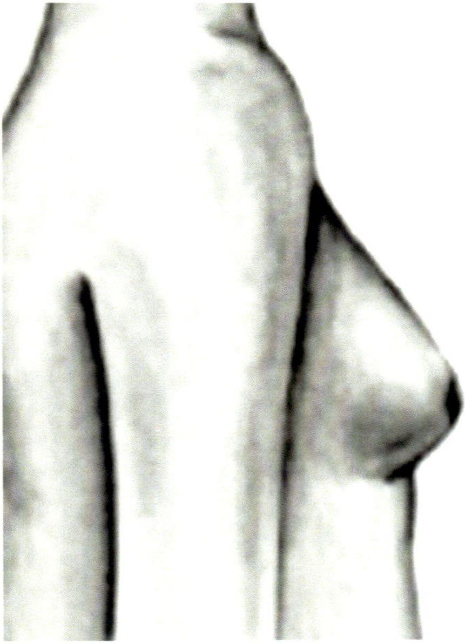

FIGURE 16.3: Stage III, the single mound enlarges.

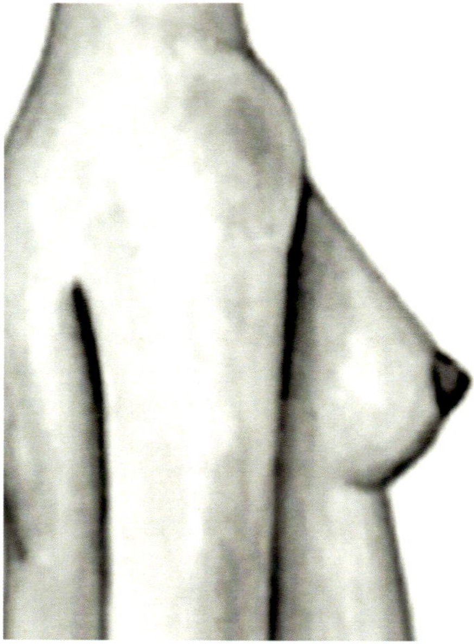

FIGURE 16.4: Stage IV, a secondary mound develops, with the nipple and areola projecting above the breast tissue.

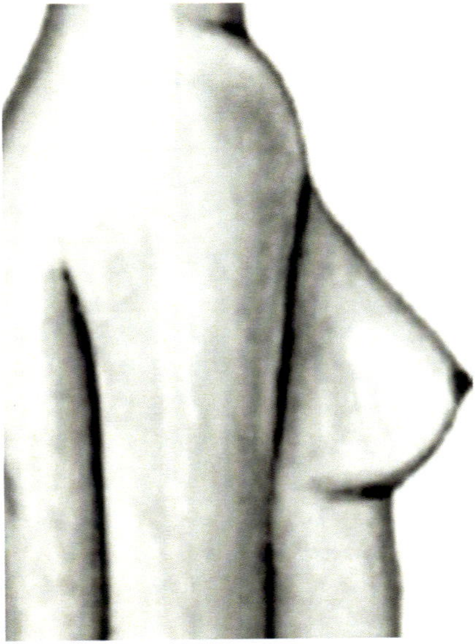

FIGURE 16.5: Stage V, the areola regresses to form a smooth contour with the rest of the breast tissue.

Tanner Staging Pubic Hair Development

- Stage I, Pre-pubertal, no pubic hair
- Stage II, Sparse, slightly pigmented, longer but still downy, straight or slightly curled hair along the labia
- Stage III, Considerably darker, coarser and more curled, sparsely over the mons

- Stage IV, Resemble the adult type, area covered is still smaller area, start to spread across the mons, no spread to medial thighs
- Stage V, adult type, darker, coarse, curled, distributed in the classic female triangle, and may be present on medial aspect of thighs.

Facial and Axillary Hair

A small amount of facial hair often develops during Tanner stage IV-V and axillary hair appears in late puberty. Detectable axillary hair will appear three to six months after beginning of appearance of pubic hair.

DEVELOPMENT OF SECONDARY SEXUAL CHARACTERISTICS IN BOYS

Tanner Staging of Pubic Hair Development

- Stage I, Prepubertal, no pubic hair
- Stage II, Sparse, slightly pigmented, longer but still downy, straight or slightly curled hair at the base of penis
- Stage III, Considerably darker, coarser and more curled, sparsely over the junction of pubes
- Stage IV, Resemble the adult type, area covered is still smaller area, no spread to medial thighs (Axillary hair start appearing)

- Stage V, Adult type, darker, coarse, curled, distributed as an inverse triangle, spreading to medial aspect of thighs, may spread up to linea alba or above base of triangle.

Tanner Staging Genital Development for Boys

- Stage I, Preadolescent. Testes, scrotum and penis are about same size
- Stage II, Scrotum and testes enlarged, penis has not enlarged, scrotal skin reddens and show a change in texture
- Stage III, Penis lengthen, further growth of testes and scrotum
- Stage IV, Breadth of penis increases, glans develops, scrotal skin darkens
- Stage V, Adult type genitalia.

Facial and Axillary Hair

Facial hair initially appears above the lip and on lower chin. Hair is seldom found on upper chin until both genitalia and pubic hair are complete. Axillary hair appears in late puberty.

ODONTOLOGICAL EXAMINATION (FIGS 16.6 AND 16.7)

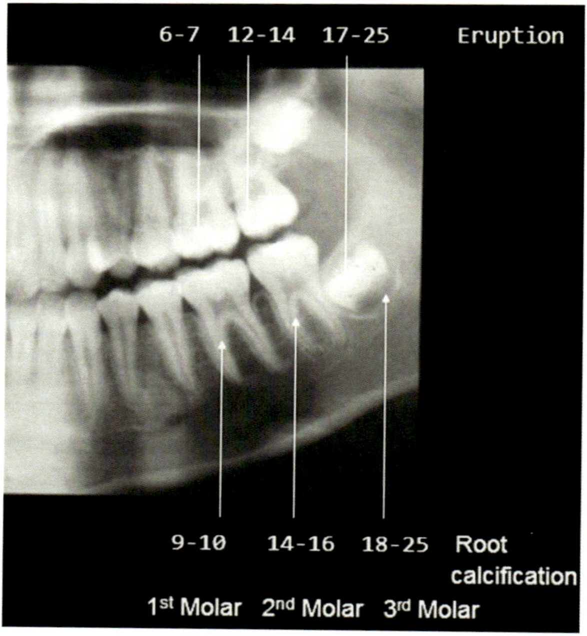

FIGURE 16.6: Odontological examination consists of noting total number of teeth in each jaw on each side, defining them as temporary or permanent and noting non-erupted or impacted teeth by physical and/or radiological examination. Eruption of permanent molars and their root calcification is very much specific in appearance.

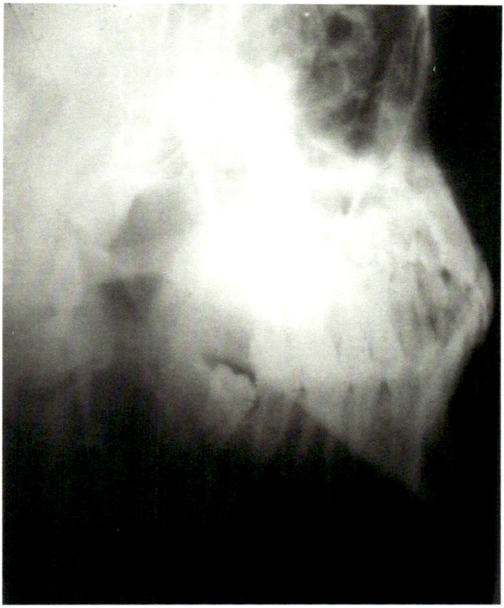

FIGURE 16.7: A lateral X-ray of skull is always helpful to determine radiological status of teeth.

RADIOLOGICAL EXAMINATION (FIGS 16.8 AND 16.9)

Radiological examination consists of advising X-ray of certain bones or joints depending on the age determined from physical and odontological examination, determining whether certain ossification centers appeared or not, if appeared whether they are fused or not and is there any ageing process.

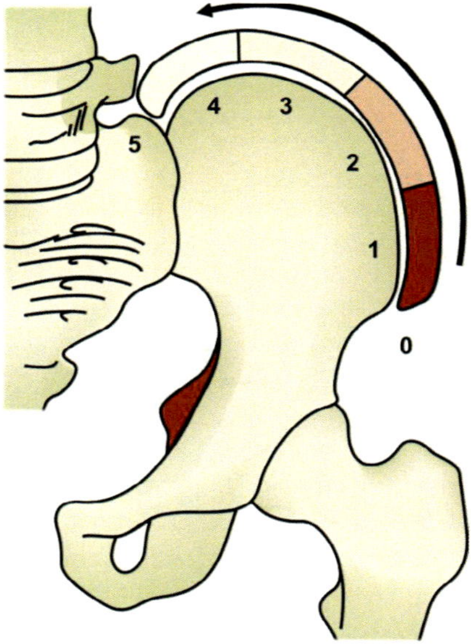

FIGURE 16.8: Risser grades 0 to 5: Centers for iliac apophysis appears at about 14 years and fusion occurs at 17 to 21 years. Grading is based on the degree of bony fusion of the iliac apophysis, from grade zero (no ossification) to grade 5 (complete bony fusion). This grading can be used for determining age from X-ray pelvis.

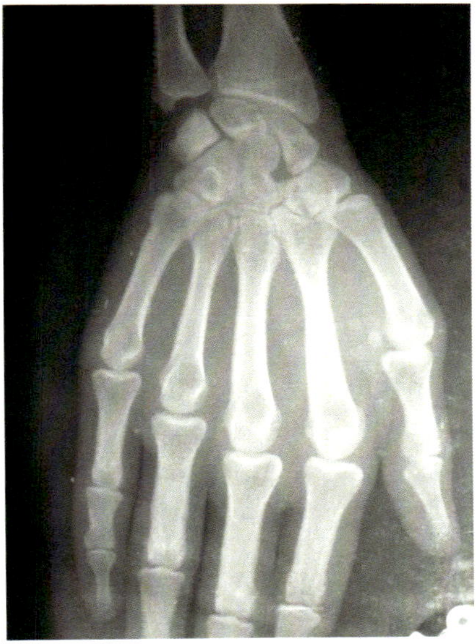

FIGURE 16.9: X-ray of radius and ulna with wrist joint and hand in a 17-year-old female. Note that the lower end of ulna completely fused with shaft (completely fuses at about 17 to 18 years of age in female) and the line of fusion is still visible between lower end of radius and shaft (completely fuses at about 18 to 19 years of age in female).

After considering history; physical, odontological and radiological findings the opinion about age of the examined person is to be formed.

Beware! Many doctors, forensic experts and even judges, lawyers and police personnel have this conception that radiological examination popularly known as "Ossification test" is the only very accurate investigation to determine age of a person. Hence it is advised by them to determine age of a person without considering physical development and odontological examination. It must be brought to the notice of the advising authority that there are many conditions and deficiencies which can delay or modify the development of bones. Hence it is very important for proper administration of justice in all such cases that the person must be examined for his/her physical development, odontological development and bone development (radiological examination) along with history recorded.

17 Examination of Physically Abused or Injured

A clinician may deal with examination of a "once physically abused victim" or "repeatedly physically abused victim". "Once physically abused" victims are usually the persons involved in scuffles, fights or interpersonal violence. However "repeatedly abused persons" are close relatives of the accused, e.g. wife, child, old aged parents or a weak person in the family.

History and explanation of causation of injury is very important and it should be noted in the report. It must be opined that the explanation and time of occurrence of injuries supplied are consistent with that of the findings rather than opining the age of injury in days and hours.

History of consumption of medicines like aspirin, anticoagulants or steroids should be ruled out as they are known to cause changes in the healing process of wound, thus affecting the calculation of age of any injury.

Age, sex, complexion, nutritional status and any disorder, allergies, bleeding disorders, etc must be considered before opining on the injury.

The data which is usually used for determination of age of injuries in morbid forensic medicine is not applicable in clinical forensic medicine.

For different types or nature of injury the related topics in the section of morbid anatomy can be referred.

EXAMINATION OF DIFFERENT INJURIES

For a clinician, management of the injury is of prime importance. However it is very important to define nature of the injury before its management. Management of the injury also depends on the site of the injury and structures involved.

Bruise (Figs 17.1 to 17.7)

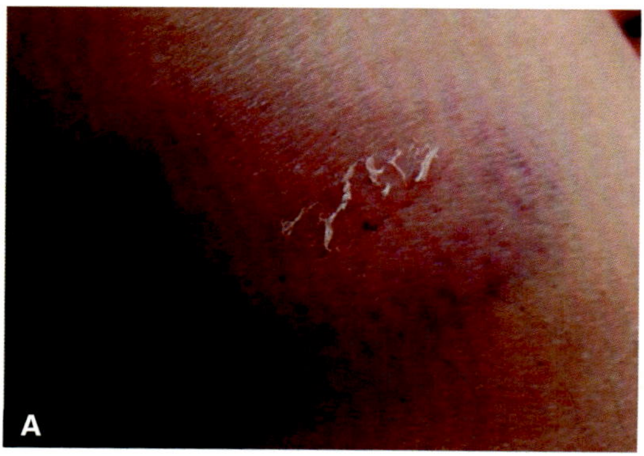

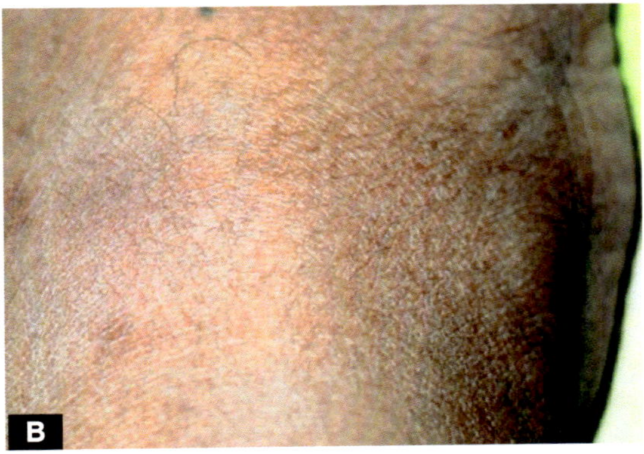

FIGURES 17.1A AND B: Bruise is the most complex and controversial type of injury. Its recognition depends on the complexion of the victim. In a dark colored victim only pain and swelling is appreciable and color changes may not be detected at all in a deep seated bruise. Compare these two bruises of about same age ~6 hours. The color is better appreciated in a fair complexioned person than that in a dark complexioned person. When the color is not appreciable at first instance, it is advisable to ask the injured to attend hospital after every 24 hours for about three to four times.

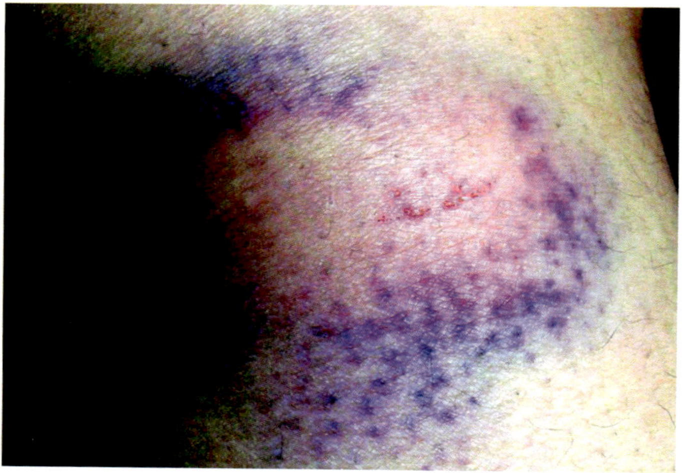

FIGURE 17.2: Color changes in the bruise are not a good marker to determine the age of a bruise. In the bruise, indicated in Figure 17.1.A, the yellow color was appreciable after 28 hours and definite yellow color was present after ~48 hours till the normal skin color became apparent on 16th day.

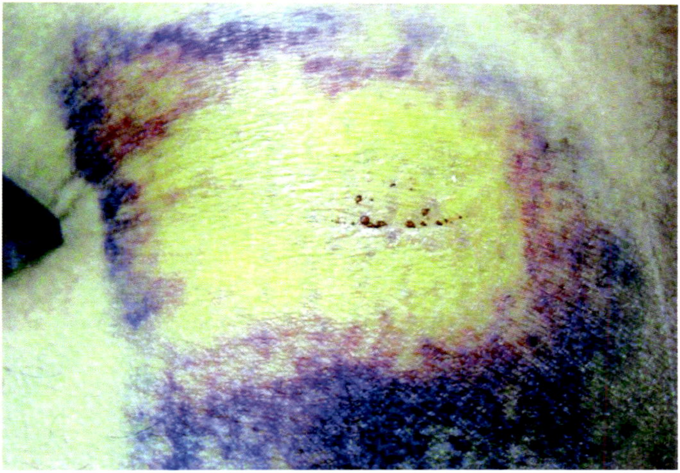

FIGURE 17.3: It is mentioned in many books that the color of bruise changes and disappears from periphery. However, this is also not the rule. As in this bruise the yellow color appeared at the central area (which was expected at periphery) and violet at periphery (which was expected at center). Age of this bruise is four days eight hours. Injuries like abrasions associated with bruise must be taken into consideration to determine age of the bruise as they show more stable changes due to healing.

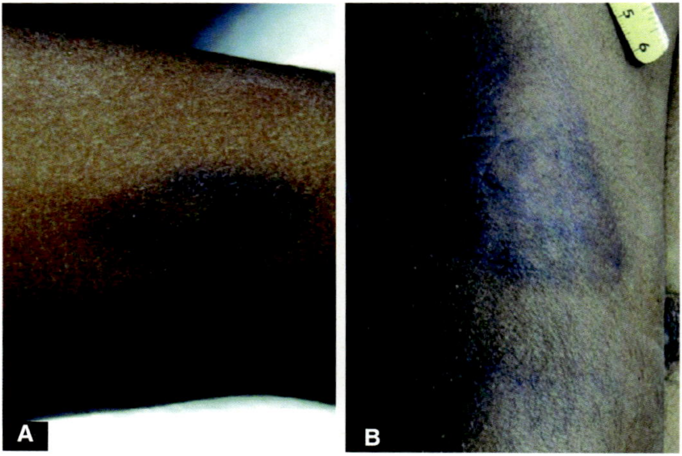

FIGURES 17.4A AND B: Certain bruises are very peculiar and possible only in physical abuse, e.g. bruises caused by pinching, squeezing, biting, holding or firm grasp. As in this case the arm was grasped and we can see the bruise depicts the impression of thumb and fingers (Age of the bruise ~16 hours).

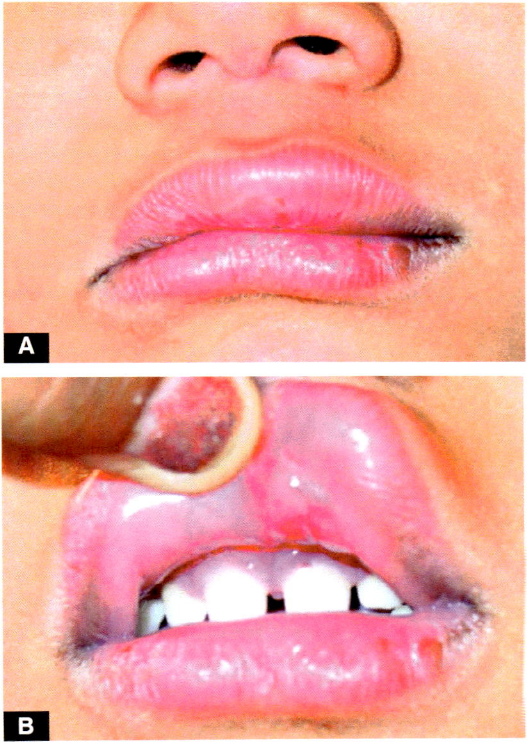

FIGURES 17.5A AND B: Bruise without any color change after ~7 hours with mucosal laceration. Such injuries can be taken as the injuries of child abuse. However the possibility of this injury caused due to fall from bed cannot be denied if the history is given like that.

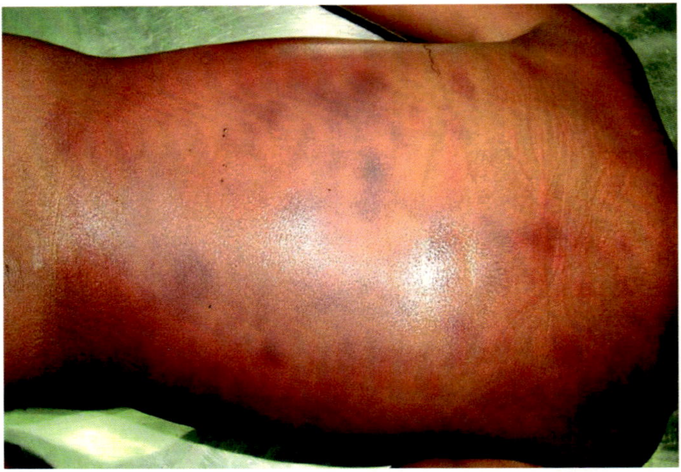

FIGURE 17.6: Multiple bruises caused by beating by stepfather in a case of child abuse. Age of all bruises is same and consistent with the history.

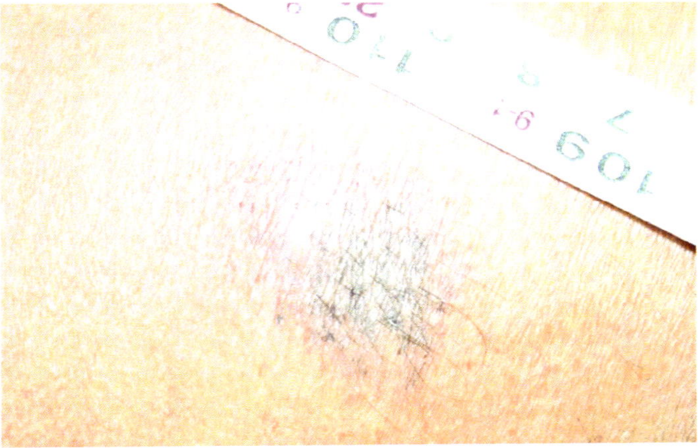

FIGURE 17.7: Beware! Skin lesions can be mistaken for bruises.

Abrasions (Figs 17.8 to 17.11)

Abrasion is very much stable injury in their healing process. Hence it can be considered as a good marker to determine age of the injury with which it is associated. However their rate of healing depends on involvement of deeper layers of skin and its size.

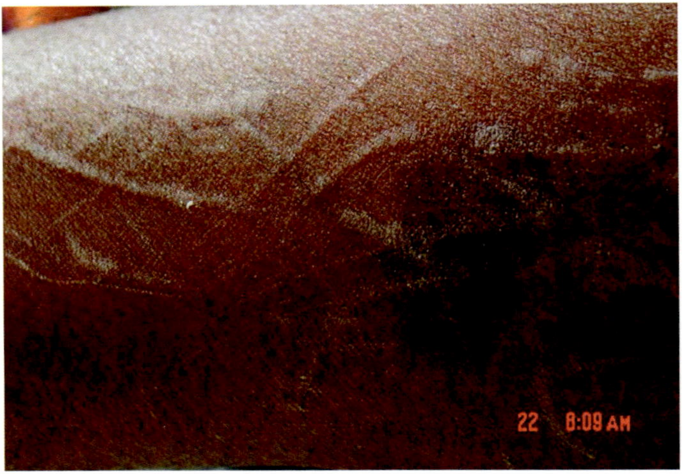

FIGURE 17.8: These are the abrasions caused by thorns. Note the swelling and no evidence of any bleeding. These types of abrasions may disappear in 2 to 3 hours without leaving any evidence on gross examination. A hand lens is a good tool for examination in such situations.

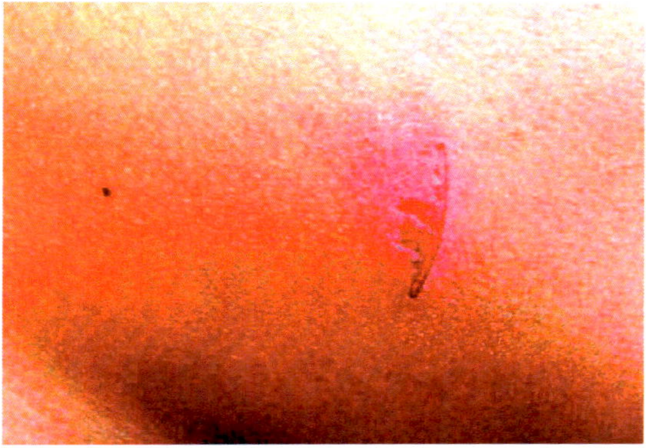

FIGURE 17.9: A day old abrasion. Note that edema and redness in the surrounding is still visible.

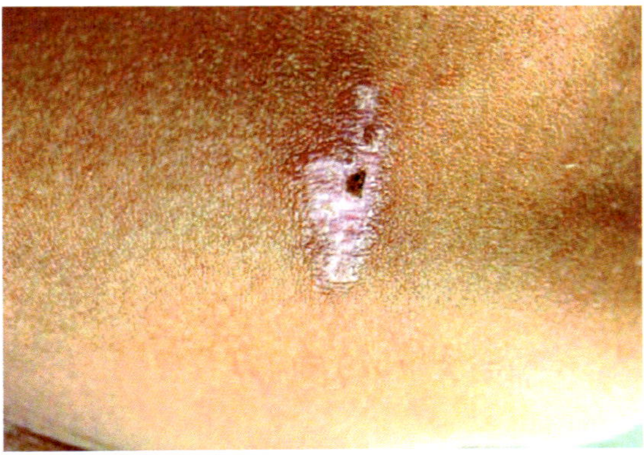

FIGURE 17.10: The same abrasion on seventh day. Note the falling scab.

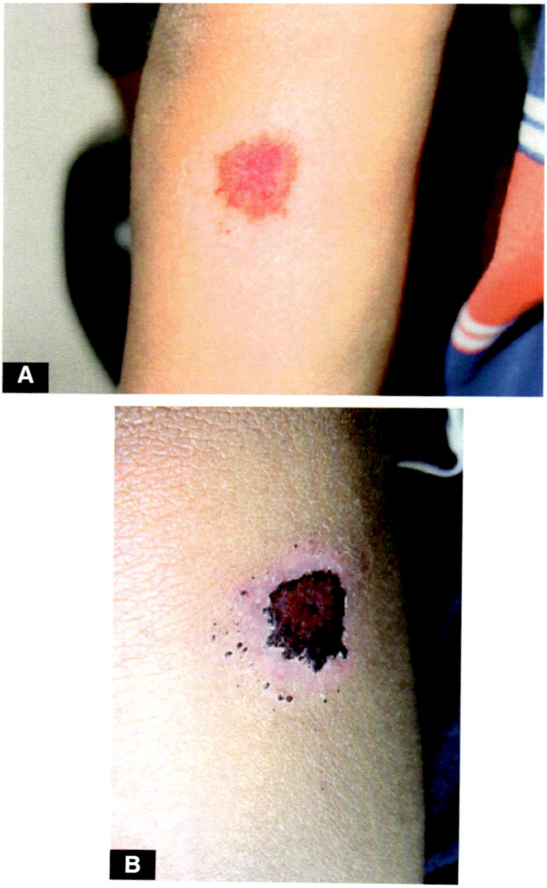

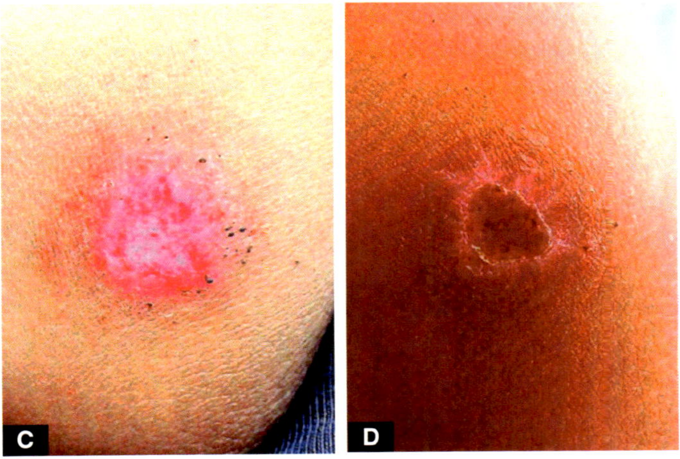

FIGURES 17.11A TO D: Sometimes repeated trauma can modify the course of healing and thus determination of age of the injury. In this case "A" is an abrasion on second day. "B" is the same abrasion on sixth day. Note the scab formation and its color red to black. "C" is the same abrasion following re-trauma on the same day. However one can notice the evidence of previous trauma in the form of peripheral small abrasions with dark black scab. "D" is the same abrasion after six days of re-trauma. Note the color of scab and compare it with scab in "B".

Lacerated, Incised and Stab Wound (Figs 17.12 to 17.14)

Defining nature of these three injuries may be sometimes difficult for the clinician. However those who are well-read in the subject forensic medicine may not find it difficult. Refer to the history or explanation given by victim and/or relatives for injury.

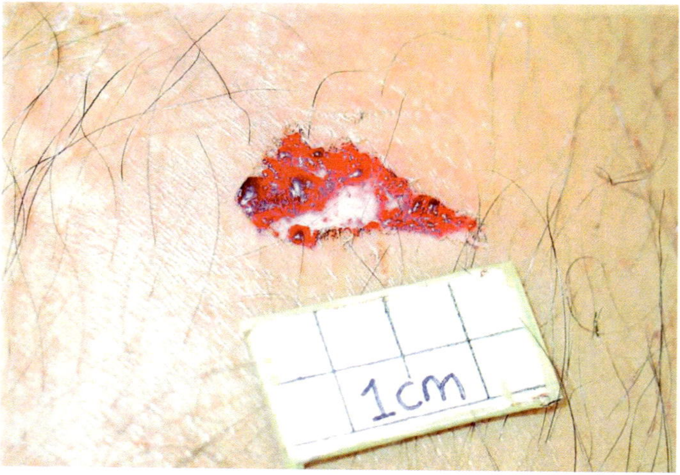

FIGURE 17.12: Laceration is usually an irregular injury present on bony area. When the doctor attends the victim, he may find that the bleeding has already stopped. While stitching the wound the clots could be found inside the wound and there are no bleeders or very few bleeders present, transverse tags of fascia, nerve or blood vessels and foreign bodies like earth particles are frequently present. Note the clotted blood at places (Age of this laceration is ~ 1 hour).

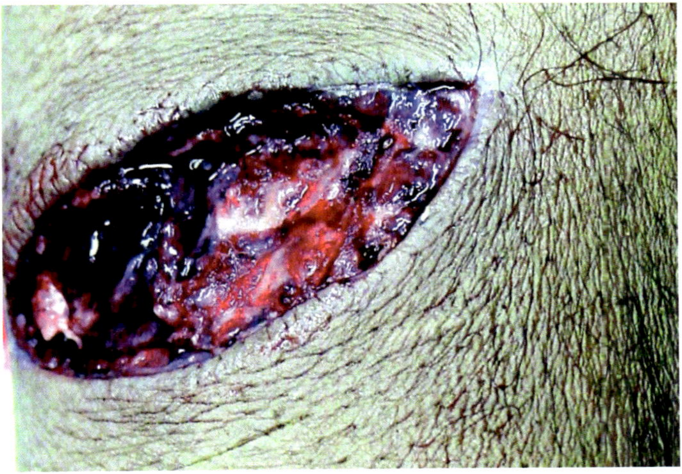

FIGURE 17.13: Incised wounds are clean cut wounds, sometimes with abraded margins if the edge of the causative weapon is rough or bruised margins if the edge of the weapon is becoming broader towards opposite end, e.g. axe. It is usually a severely bleeding wound with many bleeders depending on the site and depth of the wound without any feature of laceration. If it is present in the hairy area of body the hair in the vicinity of incised wound are found cut. The depth of this injury is always smaller than its length. This incised wound is caused by a razor. Note the edematous and inverted margins of the wound. (Age of this incised wound is ~ 1 hour).

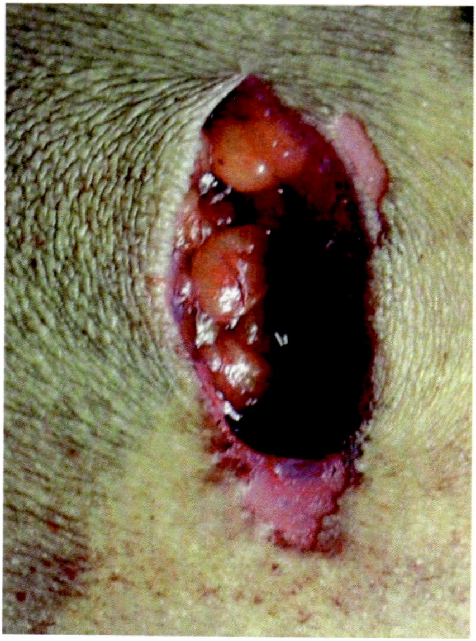

FIGURE 17.14: The peculiarity of the stab or penetrating or perforating wound is that its depth is always greater than its length. While managing these wounds the doctor should note its size, shape, margins, end and direction with the damaged internal organs on exploration of this injury. Note upper sharp end and lower rounded abraded end with left abraded margin of this stab wound. All these features will be helpful in future to identify the causative weapon (The clinician is required to decide number of stitches before stitching the wound and in that case measuring length of wound is required. The same is useful for forensic investigations).

Other Injuries (Figs 17.15 to 17.19)

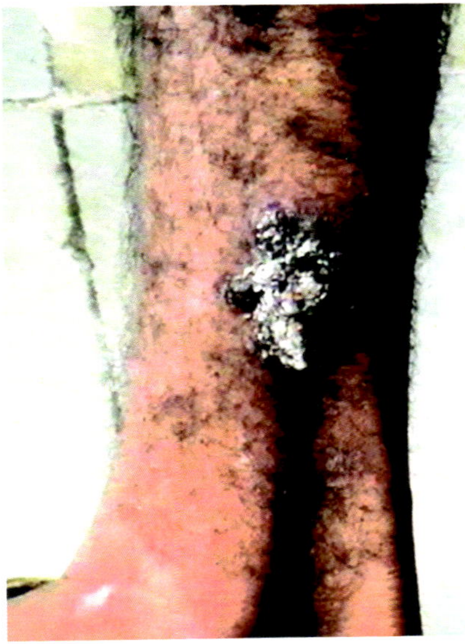

FIGURE 17.15: Many times the doctor may attend a victim with some home made medicines applied on the injuries The commonest are turmeric powder and/or slaked lime. Some time earth dust is also applied to the wound. All these elements cause modification in the appearance of injury and thus in the opinion about their age. Here the lime is applied on erosion caused by marking nut. (*Courtesy:* Dr Kailash U Zine, Associated Professor, Forensic Medicine, Govt. Medical College, Aurangabad).

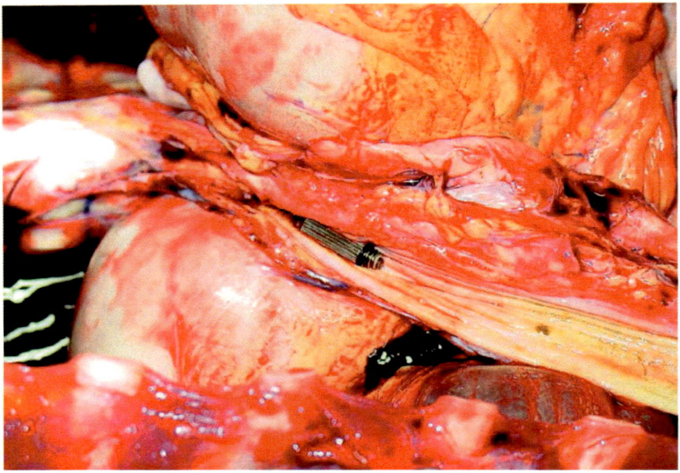

FIGURE 17.16: It is very important to mention here that every time before using any equipment, especially electrical or battery operated equipments, they must be tested for the proper electric supply and fitting. This photograph shows a bulb of laryngoscope in the esophagus (luckily not in respiratory track). The victim died during treatment of head injury.

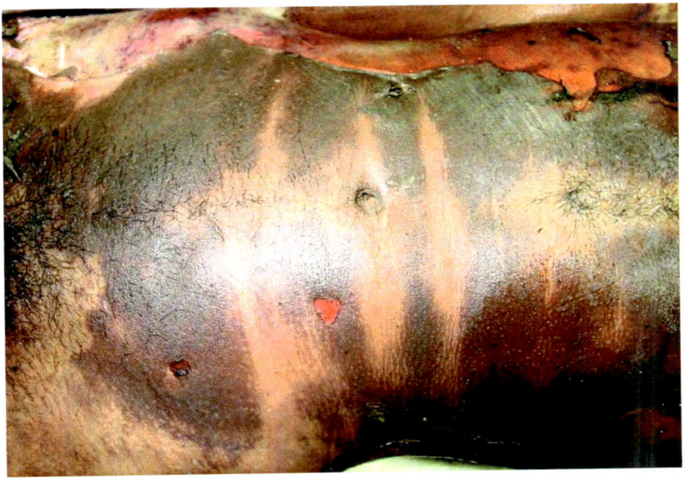

FIGURE 17.17: Burns should be mentioned with their depth, surface area involved, color, discolorations, smell, etc.

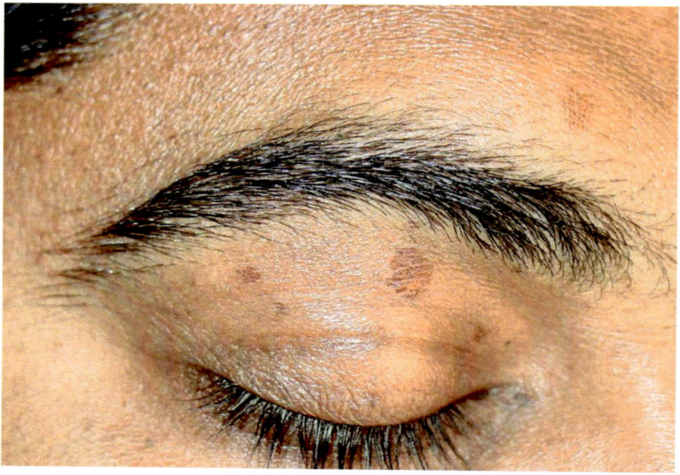

FIGURE 17.18: Scalds are very peculiar injuries. This photograph shows accidental burns by hot oil drops.

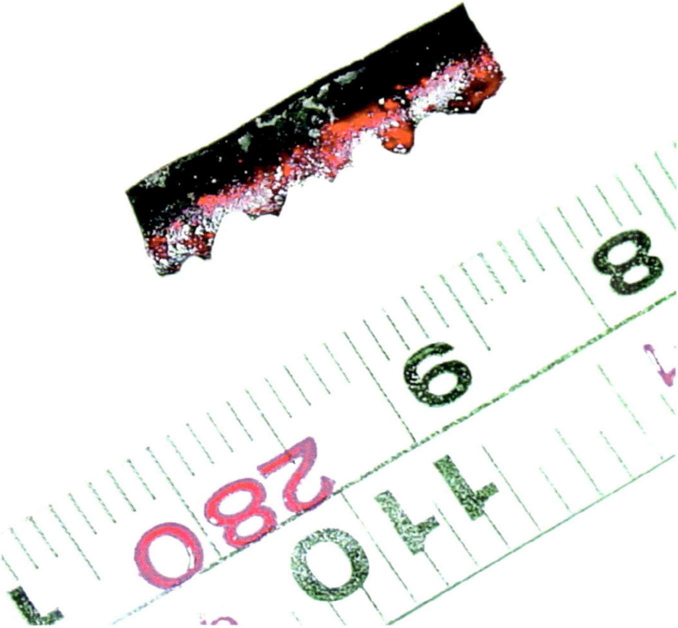

FIGURE 17.19: Foreign body if any removed during managing a wound should be preserved without washing in a gauze piece and cardboard box.

SITE OF INJURY (FIGS 17.20 TO 17.25)

The site of injury should be mentioned with respect to two anatomical landmarks.

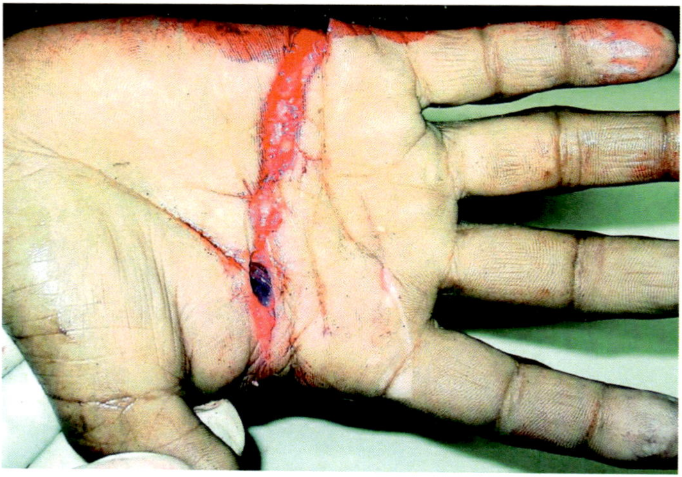

FIGURE 17.20: Deep incised wound on palm indicate a defense injury while holding weapon in defense.

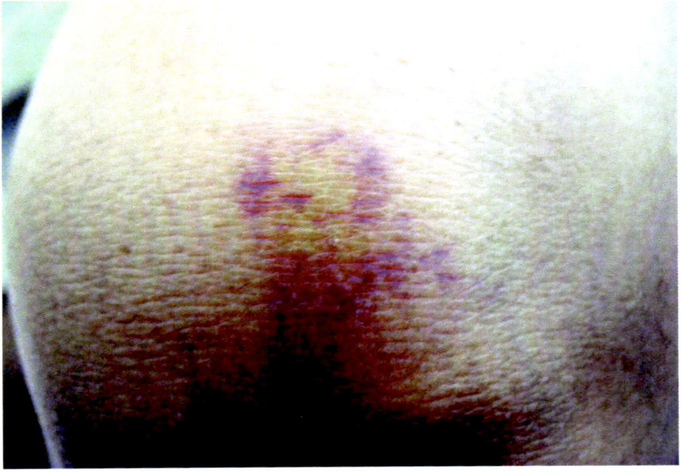

FIGURE 17.21: Bruise and abrasions to knee are commonly found in simple fall. Note extravasation of blood is comparatively more in lines of Langer.

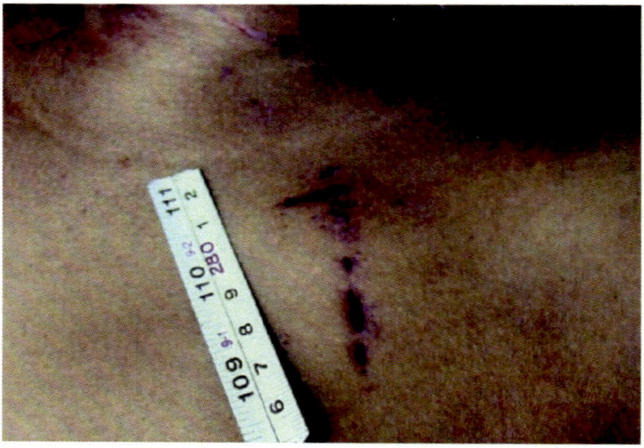

FIGURE 17.22: Scratches around neck or peri-clavicular region indicate scuffle.

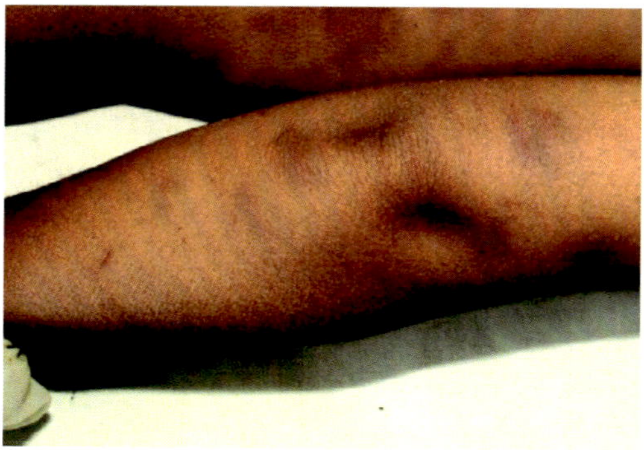

FIGURE 17.23: Multiple discoid bruise around wrist, forearm, elbow or arm indicate forceful holding or firm griping by the accused.

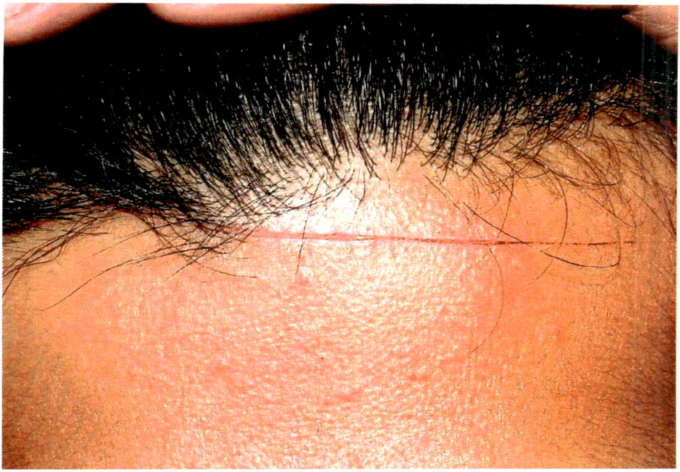

FIGURE 17.24: This linear scratch abrasion is caused by glass coated kite-string (Manja). It is one of the common accidental injuries found in kite flying season in India. The common sites of these injuries are where the kite-string gets entangled.

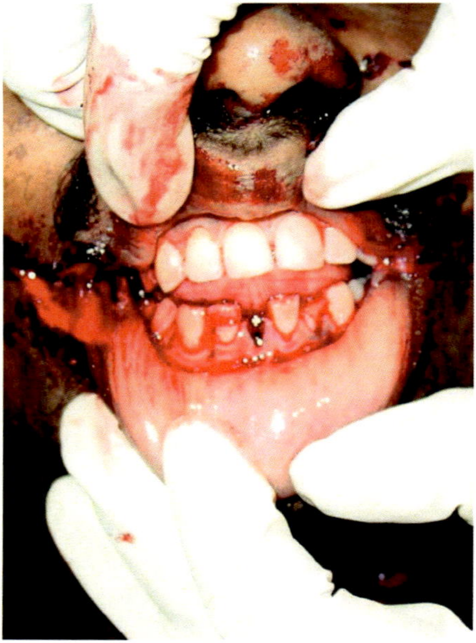

FIGURE 17.25: Cutting tongue or injuries caused in trying to cut tongue is an intentional injury usually indicating previous verbal abuse by the victim.

GRIEVOUS HURT OR NOT

In Indian legal context it is essential to define whether the examined injury is grievous or not. There is no legal definition of simple injury; hence the injury can be grievous or non-grievous. The term simple injury is almost always taken so simply that it seems that the injury has no medico-legal significance. Only those injuries, which are mentioned in section 320 of Indian Penal Code are grievous and all other injuries are not grievous (do not call them as a simple injury).

Following hurts are designated as grievous hurt as per Sec 320 IPC

1. *Emasculation:* meaning by taking away the masculinity or maleness. This clause is applicable only to males.
2. Permanent privation of sight of either eye.
3. Permanent privation of hearing of either ear.
   In 2 and 3, the words permanent and privation are very important. The privation must be permanent. Many Indian textbooks mention the meaning of these clauses as permanent loss of sight or hearing. However, the word privation means "the act of depriving somebody of something". Loss is not a punishable act but the act of depriving somebody of something is punishable by law. It is always advisable to give opinion on this type of injury after complete healing and investigation when the injury seems to be minor.
4. *Privation of any member or joint:* Member of the body means limb or organ with a specific function.

5. *Destruction or permanent impairing of powers of any member or joint:* The impairment is supposed to be permanent. Hence it is advisable that opinion about these types of injuries should be given after complete healing of the injuries.
6. *Permanent disfiguration of the head or face:* The injury to head and face are included in this clause. They must cause permanent disfiguration.
7. Fracture or dislocation of a bone or tooth.
8. *Any hurt which endangers life or which causes the victim to be in severe bodily pain, or unable to follow his ordinary pursuits for a period of 20 days:* When the injury endangers life or put into risk of death OR when it is proved that the victim was suffering from severe bodily pain or unable to do his daily work, e.g. getting out of bed, cleaning, taking bath, preparing and eating meal, etc. for the period of 20 days.

MAKING REMARK

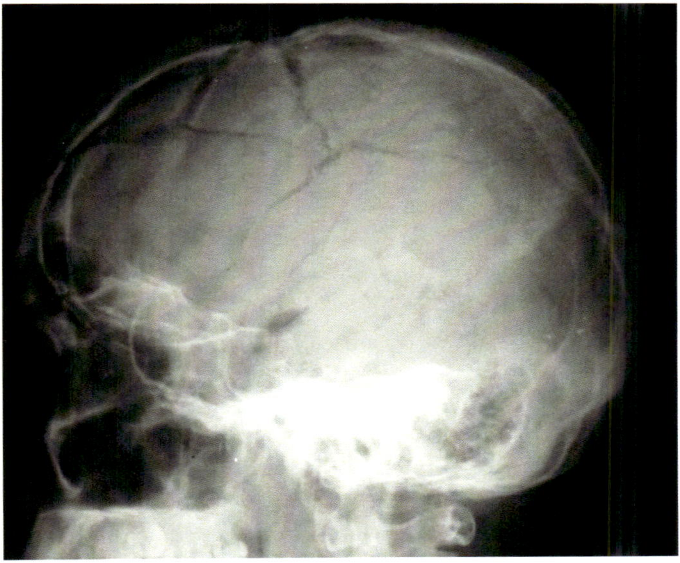

FIGURE 17.26: It must be mentioned in the report itself if the second or subsequent examinations are necessary OR the radiological examination is necessary before making an opinion OR when opinions will be given after complete healing or certain medical investigations if necessary. Externally non-grievous head injury may become grievous on X-ray skull.

18 Examination of Weapons

A weapon is a device designed to injure or kill. There are two types of weapons which a doctor could come across. The first one is a weapon which fits exactly in the definition of weapon (Fig. 18.1) i.e. it has no other use than to injure or kill, e.g. sword, pistol, dagger, etc. While others are the tools or objects used as a weapon of offence (Fig. 18.7) e.g. kitchen knife, shaving blade, axe, etc.

Receiving the weapon of offence with requisition and queries is a frequent activity after autopsy or examination of abused or injured. Before accepting any article from the investigating authority it must be verified that whether it is properly packed, labeled and sealed. The seal on the packet must be verified by tallying it with a sample of seal on the requisition or query letter. If any discrepancy is found then it should be brought to the notice and returned to the police personnel who brought it. If everything is found correct then such note should be made along with the receipt of the requisition or query and the article.

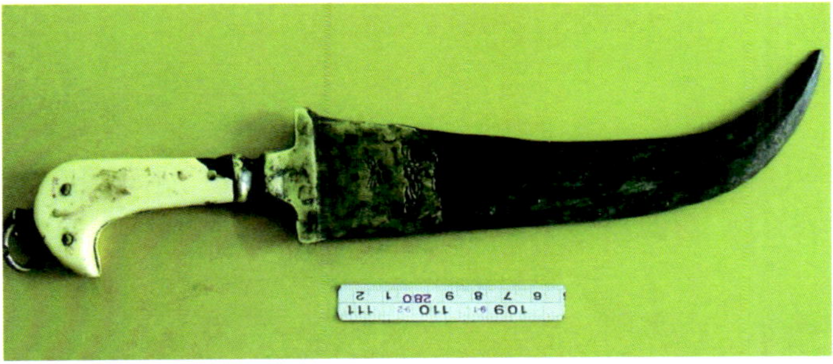

FIGURE 18.1: Dagger

PREPARING REPORT

A. Name of the weapon should be the local name of the weapon, e.g. Kurhad instead of Axe or Bhala instead of spear.

B. *Kind of the weapon:* There is no universal classification of weapons. However they can be grouped in different kinds of objects

   i Blunt (light or heavy) (flexible/hard/rough)

   ii Cutting edged (sharp cutting/rough cutting/serrated/blunt, etc.) (light or heavy)

   iii Pointed (sharp/blunt/rounded/curved, etc).

   Combination of i, ii, and iii is a commonest occurrence.

   Examples: Figures 18.2 to 18.4.

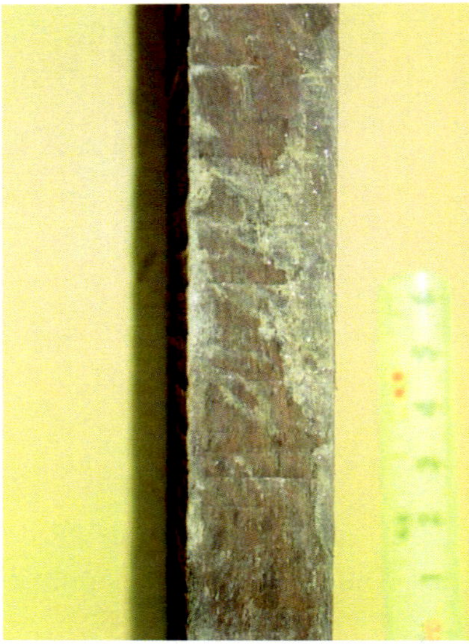

FIGURE 18.2: This is a wooden plank; a hard blunt heavy kind of weapon. But the object has rough margins also.

C. *Dangerous or not dangerous:* In India, the definition of dangerous weapon can be extracted from section 324 and 326 of Indian Penal Code as "any instrument which can be used for cutting, stabbing or shooting or when it is used as a weapon of offence is likely to cause death". There is no definition of simple or not dangerous weapon given by law. Many times the

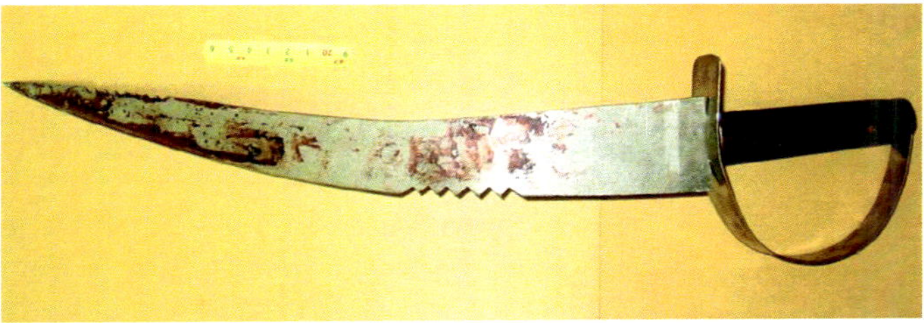

FIGURE 18.3: This is a dagger with sharp pointed blade with sharp cutting and serrated edges.

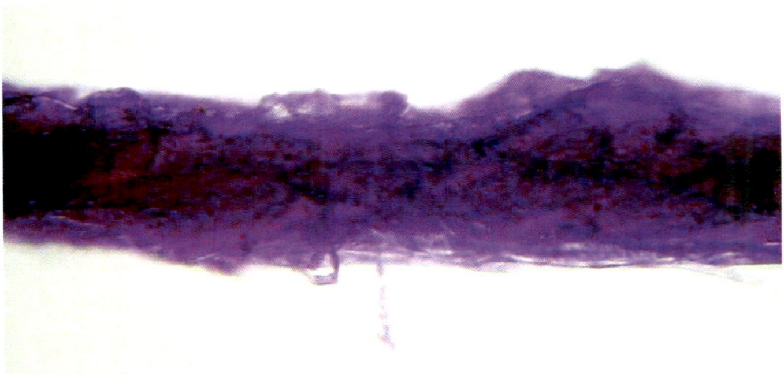

FIGURE 18.4: A microscopic view of “Manja” a glass coated kite-string showing cutting edge of the ground glass adherent to the kite-string. It is a flexible sharp cutting light object (X100 unstained).

weapon for examination is non-dangerous, except in some contexts they can be dangerous. Hence it should be described in detail about such weapons, e.g. the wooden plank is a non-dangerous weapon except when it is used with substantial force on head, it can cause fracture of skull and subsequent death. In such a situation the wooden plank becomes a dangerous weapon.

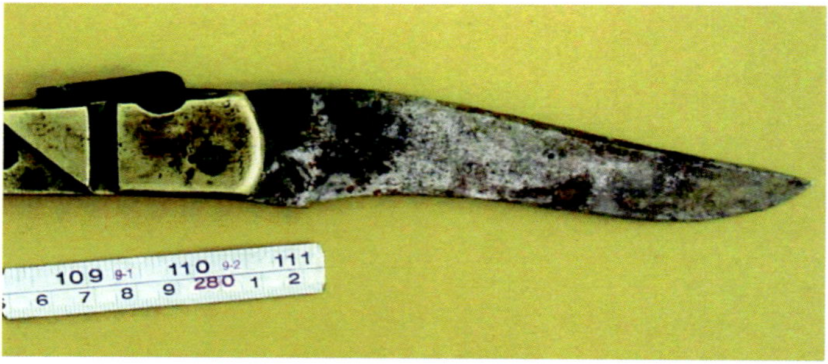

FIGURE 18.5: This is a blade of a knife locally called as "Rampuri". Mentioning curvature of the blade is very important as its point and convex curvature can cause a stab with both ends sharp although only one margin of the blade is sharp cutting and other is blunt.

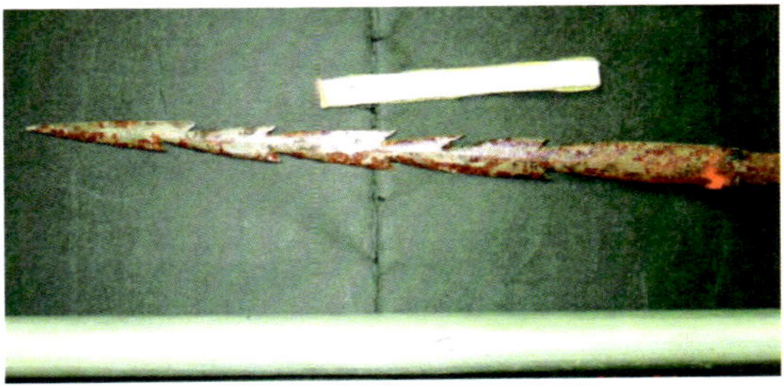

FIGURE 18.6: When the blade has serrated margins with angulations towards handle then such weapons are known to cause stab wounds with protrusion of internal tissue or viscera. The sheath of the weapon is also shown in this photograph. When the sheath is present with the weapon its complete description should be given which should contain data of its length, thickness, texture and presence of any stain, prints or foreign bodies especially on its inner surface.

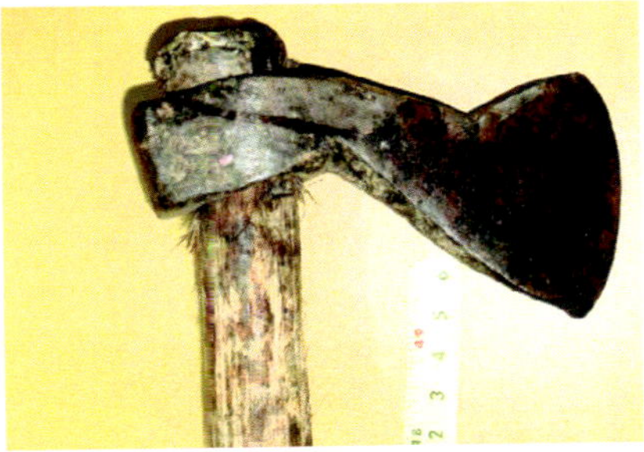

FIGURE 18.7: An axe is a weapon which has blade without point. Hence the commonest possible injuries are chop and incised wounds. Note the dried blood stain.

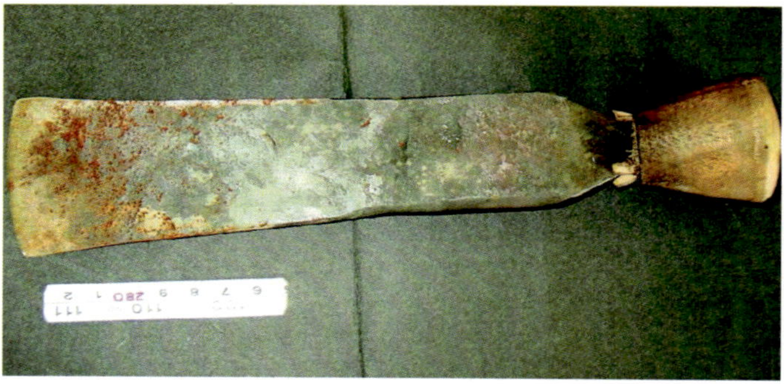

FIGURE 18.8: A similar weapon without point is a leather cutter (this instrument is commonly used by persons involved in the business of repairing or making shoes). A similar instrument is also used in the work related to wood carving. The commonest injury is a chop wound or stab wound with cutting of underlying bone.

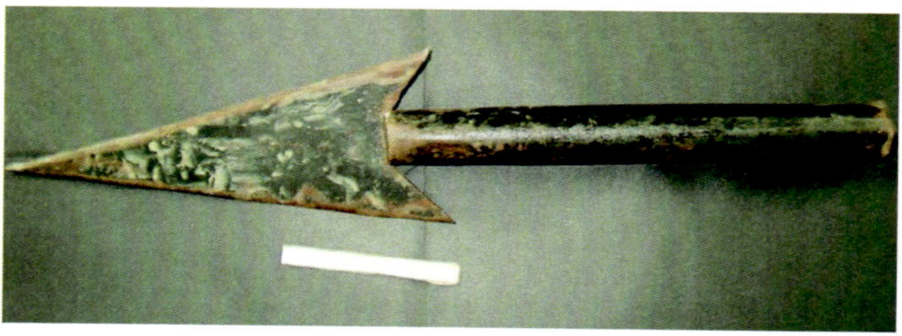

FIGURE 18.9: Blade or head of spear is a weapon which commonly causes stab or glancing cuts. Glancing cuts are the incised wounds usually found on the rounded contour of the body especially on the outer surface.

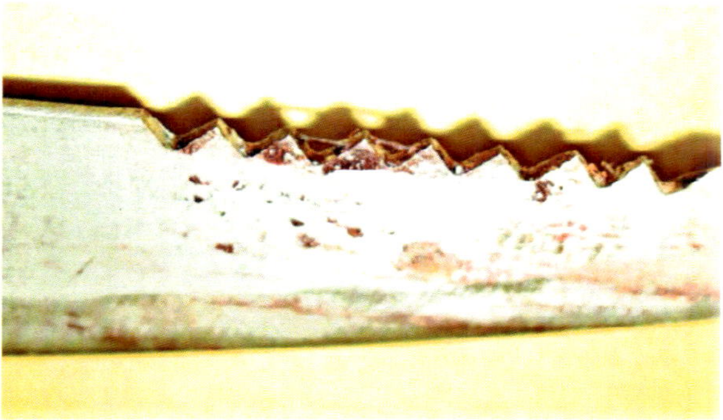

FIGURE 18.10: Examination of serrated or damaged edges of the blade may reveal presence of tissue, threads or other foreign body from the victim.

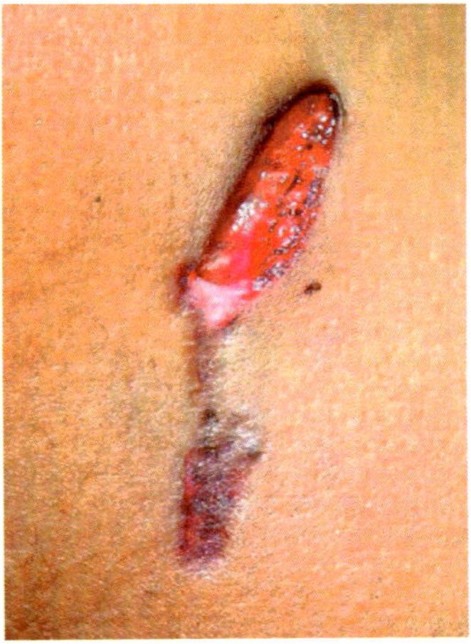

FIGURE 18.11: Joint between handle and blade is also an important area as it may damage the surrounding area of the stab wound if the blade of the weapon is completely thrust in the body.

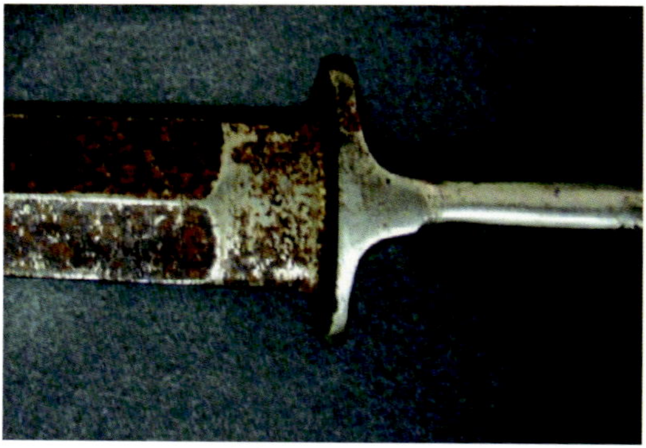

FIGURE 18.12: When the joint is of fixed type it is either with hilt or without hilt. If the weapon possesses hilt then it may cause contusion or abrasion around stab as a hilt mark when the blade of the weapon is impaled with force up to hilt.

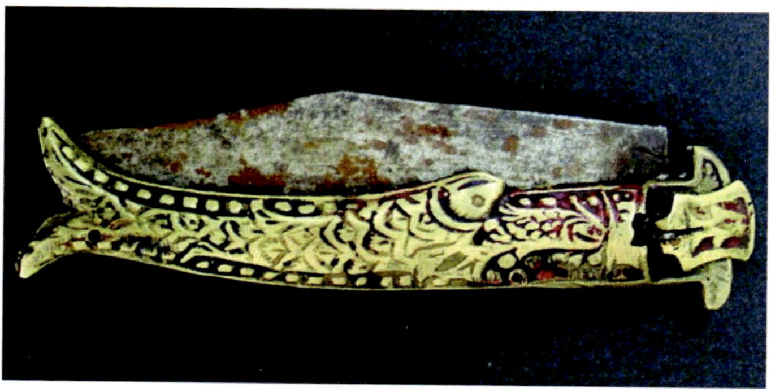

FIGURE 18.13: When the joint is of hinge type then it may be with lock system or without lock system.

D. *Description of the weapon:* There is no specific format for description of the weapon for examination e.g. if a heavy stone is a weapon of offence then it can be described in its maximum length, breadth and thickness; presence of any sharp edges; and its weight.

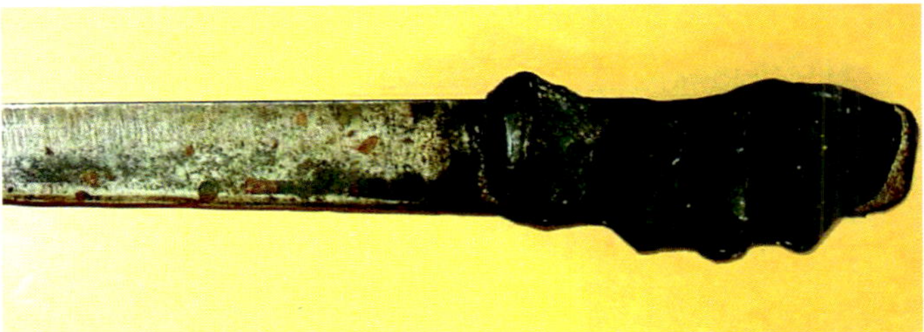

FIGURE 18.14: This weapon has a very peculiar grip made-up of an adhesive material usually used to seal the leakages in the water pipes (M-Seal™). This grip gives exact dimensions of the makers griping palm.

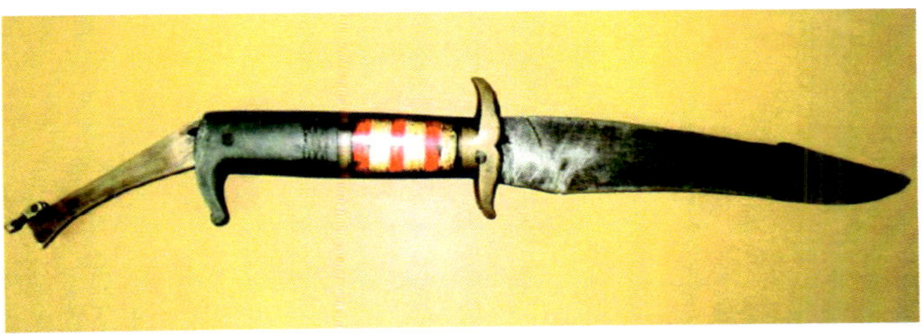

FIGURE 18.15: Sometimes a part of lock system may be present at the rare end of the handle.

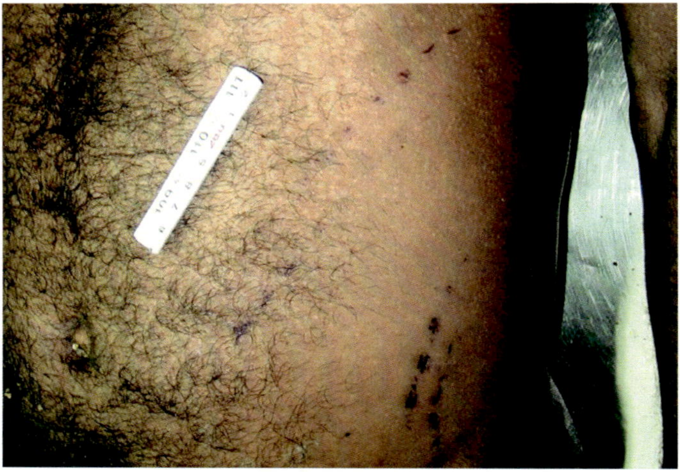

FIGURE 18.16: If the imprint injuries are found on the body then they should be carefully recorded and if possible photographed with a measuring scale. After receipt of the weapon the injuries should be compared with the class and individual characteristics of the weapon.

However many weapons can be described in the form of their blade, handle and joint between them.

Blade is an important part of a weapon as it imparts some peculiarity to the injury. Its description should contain details about its length, breadth, thickness, margins and point. Other description includes roughness of blade, stains, prints or foreign body if any.

The details of handle or grip should be mentioned in the form of its length, breadth or circumference and texture. It is the most decorated part of the weapon. Sometimes the name of owner may be found on this part.

OPINION

Opinion about injuries possible by the examined weapon should be formed on the basis of kind of weapon and its peculiarities. Commonest injury should form the first opinion and rarest injury should be mentioned with their possibility and the methodology by which they are possible.

The weapon must be signed on the unstained area to identify it in future as and when required.

If any foreign body is found adherent to the weapon it should be covered by a transparent adhesive tape to avoid its lose in further transaction and a note about the same should be mentioned in the report.

After proper packing and sealing the weapon should be handed over to the police personnel on duty by taking receipt of the same.

It is always advisable to send the weapon to forensic science lab for further examination.

19 Examination in Sexual Offences

Three types of patients can be examined under this topic:

1. Female victim of sexual offence
2. Male victim of sexual offence and
3. Male accused of sexual offence.

The questions to be answered after examination are:

1. Is there any finding suggestive of sexual intercourse?
2. Is there any sign of struggle?
3. Are the clinical findings compatible with the history of incident recorded?
4. What is the co-relation of reports of preserved samples from forensic science laboratory with clinical findings?

Medical examination should be carried out without any delay. Sympathetic behavior should be maintained. Unnecessary verbal and written comments should be avoided. There are many myths about sexual offences. The examination should be conducted in a well lighted room. The victim or accused should be requested to remove their clothes on a clean white hospital bed sheet or paper so that any material falling on the bed-sheet or paper can be collected for further examination. Blood should be collected for toxicological analysis as well as for blood grouping. Swab should be collected from buccal cavity if there is history of oral coitus.

EXAMINATION OF FEMALE VICTIM OF SEXUAL OFFENCE

History of incidence of sexual offence in respect to time and place with details like whether she was intoxicated or in her senses, if there is delay in reporting the incidence then the reason for the same, whether she struggled or cried for help, if no then why not, whether complete clothes were removed or not, if removed then by whom, whether she felt penetration, was it painful, what was the relative position of accused during the incidence, whether she passed urine or stool, whether she had washed her genitalia or taken bath, whether she changed the clothes, onset of puberty and last menstruating period, whether she was menstruating at the time of incident, is she habitual to sexual intercourse, if yes, since when, has she delivered baby, if yes then when.

In general examination the built and mental status of the victim should be recorded. Noting details of type of dress and make-up are important with its damage. If the victim is wearing the same clothing at the time of incidence then they should be examined after removal for damages, stains and foreign bodies. Their details must be mentioned in the report. The clothes should be properly signed, packed in a paper bag and then in a plastic bag with rents, sealed and sent to forensic science lab for further examination along with other articles and samples. The body surface should be examined for any stains, foreign bodies and injuries. The injuries should be recorded in the format of injury certificate, i.e. its nature, site, shape, direction, age, dimensions, etc. Nails should be examined for damages and foreign bodies. Nail clippings should be collected at this time. Foreign bodies, if any found on body, should be collected in a sterile bottle or paper bag depending on the type of material. Stains if found on body surface should be collected by a moist swab which should be air dried after preparing a smear on clean glass slide and preserved in a sterile bottle or test tube for further investigation. Every article should be numbered and its site from where it is collected should be mentioned. Systemic examination should not be missed.

The local examination includes examination of genitalia, perineum and anus. Pubic hair should be examined for matting; matted area of pubic hair should be cut by scissors and collected in a paper bag. Collect any avulsed or foreign hair found by combing the pubic hair. Precaution must be taken so that the gloves do not get contaminated. Use different sterile swabs moistened by distilled water for collecting specimens from different area of genitalia. Examination of area should be followed by collecting sample. Start from outside. First swab should be collected from vulva, second from peri-vaginal area and labia majora, third from labia minora and vaginal opening, fourth from vaginal canal, fifth from peri-anal and anal opening and sixth from deep anal area. From every swab a smear should be prepared on a clean glass slide and all slides should be examined for sperm. All these areas should be examined for injuries like lacerations, abrasions, bruise etc. It must be remembered that there are always injuries to the vagina when proper position is not acquired during sexual intercourse by the female which is very frequent in cases of sexual offence. Redness due to itching is almost always associated with abrasions which can be appreciated by examining the area with hand lens.

EXAMINATION OF MALE VICTIM OF SEXUAL OFFENCE (BUGGERY)

History and general examination is same as described for female victim.

Some points are to be added in the history like whether he is a homosexual, if yes then active or passive or act as both. Clothes should be examined for fecal stains.

In the local examination penis and scrotum must be examined for injuries. A swab must be collected from buccal cavity if the victim gives history of oral coitus. Swabs should be collected from peri-anal area for semen or lubricant, second swab from anal opening and third from deep anal canal. Smears should be prepared from all swabs and examined for sperm. At this point it must be remembered that skin of anal opening is very delicate and sensitive. Penetrating any object including penis cause laceration, bruising and/or severe edema of that skin. This could not occur even with passing hard stool. Proctoscopic examination is advisable after collection of samples.

EXAMINATION OF ACCUSED OF SEXUAL OFFENCE (RAPE AND BUGGERY)

History, general examination and local examination is the same as described for female and male victim.

Local examination should consist of examination of penis for any staining, soiling and injury. The pubic hair should be examined for matting, avulsed or foreign hair. Prepuce, frenulum and shaft of penis should be examined for injuries and swabs should be collected from urethra, glans prepuce, coronal sulcus and shaft of penis. Presence of smegma should be noticed. Any disease or abnormality of the penis, scrotum and testes should be noticed.

Opinion should be based on the clinical findings, history given and reports from forensic science lab. It should fulfill the objects of examination. It must be remembered that the term "Rape" is a legal term and not a medical term. Hence it must not be included in the opinion. It should also be remembered that there will be no signs of struggle if the victim was unconscious or intoxicated or unable to understand the act.

20 Examination of Drunkenness

Alcohol consumption is popularly referred to consumption of country or foreign branded liquor which contains ethyl alcohol in different concentration. However methyl alcohol is usually used in adulterated liquor.

History is a very important part to be considered before opining.

History of drinking time, quantity of alcohol consumed, illness, medicine; diabetes; mouth wash; injury; any other intoxicant.

In the examination following points should be noted along with general examination:

Attitude	Whether he is well-mannered/excited/amusing or funny/talkative/without worries or responsibility/sleepy/co-operative/without care or interest/opposing/over-confident/fighting/insulting/any other finding